EAT WELL,
LOSE WEIGHT,
WHILE BREASTFEEDING

EAT WELL, LOSE WEIGHT, WHILE BREASTFEEDING

The Complete Nutrition
Book for Nursing Mothers

EILEEN BEHAN, R.D.

BALLANTINE BOOKS   NEW YORK

A Ballantine Books Trade Paperback

Copyright © 1992, 2006 by Eileen Behan, R.D.

Published in the United States by Ballantine Books,
an imprint of The Random House Publishing Group,
a division of Random House, Inc., New York.

BALLANTINE and colophon are registered trademarks
of Random House, Inc.

Originally published in a different form and in paperback
in the United States by Villard Books, an imprint of
The Random House Publishing Group, a division of
Random House, Inc., in 1992.

ISBN 978-0-345-49259-3

Library of Congress Cataloging-in-Publication Data

Behan, Eileen.
Eat well, lose weight, while breastfeeding : the complete nutrition book for nursing
mothers / Eileen Behan R.D.—[Rev. ed.]
p. cm.
"A Ballantine Books trade paperback"
Includes bibliographical references and index.
ISBN 978-0-345-49259-3
1. Breastfeeding. 2. Mothers—Nutrition. 3. Lactation—Nutritional aspects.
4. Reducing diets. I. Title.

RJ216.B34 2006
613.2'69—dc22   2006048358

Printed in the United States of America

www.ballantinebooks.com

2 4 6 8 9 7 5 3

Book design by JoAnne Metsch

In memory of my father, John M. Behan,
and my mother, Elizabeth J. Behan

To David, Sarah, and Emily.

We did it again. Thank you.

ACKNOWLEDGMENTS

To my mother, Sharon, Sheila, and Kevin, thanks for your continuous encouragement. Trish Cronan, Brad Lavigne, as always you are a steadfast source of support. Judith Paige, Marilyn DeSimone, Madeleine Walsh, as friends and competent nutritionists, you continue to help me refine my idea. I'd like to thank Ms. Ana Ortiz for efficient and accurate nutritional analysis of menus, and Susan Yorstin, thanks again for proofreading. Ms. Susan Cotter, Jennifer Quirk, and Kathleen Beede, thank you for your comments and development of the exercise program.

I would like to thank the following nutrition and lactation experts who generously gave their time to read all or part of this before it went to print: Nancy F. Butte, Ph.D., Children's Nutrition Research Center, Houston, Texas; Bette Crase of the Center for Breastfeeding Information at La Leche League International; Kathyryn Dewey, Ph.D., professor, Department of Nutrition, University of California, Davis, California; Lois Jovanovic-Peterson, M.D., senior scientist, Sansum Medical Research Foundation, Santa Barbara, California; Ruth A. Lawrence, M.D., professor of pediatrics, obstetrics, and gynecology, University of Rochester Medical Center, Rochester, New York; Susan Luke, M.S., R.D., nutritionist–sports medicine, Boston, Massachusetts; Arnold Schecter, M.D., professor of preventive medicine, State University of New York, Binghamton, New York.

At Villard Books I would like to thank Emily Bestler and her assistant, Tom Fiffer, for working patiently with me. I am also thankful to the others at Villard who contributed significantly to this book: Richard Aquan, Nancy Inglis, and Amy Ryan. Thank you to Johanna Bowman and Rebecca Shapiro at Ballantine for their skillful revisions. I would also like to thank Patricia Martin for typing the revised manuscript.

To Allison Acker and Carol Mann, once again you both saw possibilities in my idea.

CONTENTS

INTRODUCTION
Spring 2007

A lot has changed in the world since the first edition of *Eat Well, Lose Weight, While Breastfeeding* was published in 1992. The main principle—that breastfeeding is the undisputed best way to feed babies—has, however, remained a constant. Research continues to confirm the tremendous health benefits of breastfeeding for both mother and child.

Though eating well remains a fundamental principle to a satisfying nursing experience, there are no absolute "food rules." Women from around the world eat a variety of foods and breastfeed successfully. When it comes to weight loss, the slow and steady approach is advised. *Eat Well, Lose Weight, While Breastfeeding* survived the no-fat diets of the 1990s and the no-carb craze popular in the early years of the twenty-first century. Neither extreme led to permanent weight loss. In fact, the opposite occurred. After thirty years as a nutrition educator, I have learned that those who are successful with permanent weight control are the women who adopt a healthy lifestyle.

This edition updates the content of the earlier book and includes information on new trends and concerns. The fundamental message, however, remains the same: eat well and you will lose weight and be healthy. Give your body the food it needs, allow time to care for and nurse your baby, and both of you will have a satisfying breastfeeding experience.

There is a new issue added to this revised edition. The rise in obesity among children as well as adults required the inclusion of chapter 12. In 1992, 25 percent of adult women were considered overweight. Now it is 50 percent of women. In this section you will read what to do after you stop nursing and your baby is on solid foods. Many family health specialists now describe our food environment as "toxic" because it promotes processed foods, highly advertised snacks, and harried meals that make it almost impossible to eat well and control weight. Planning family meals that are structured and predictable and contain wholesome food is the antidote to our less than perfect food environment. This edition provides me with an opportunity to offer some guidance in the area of introducing foods and establishing routines that I believe will lay the foundation for your family's meal and eating routines for years to come.

Eileen Behan

INTRODUCTION
First Edition

"Y ou should know better!" Those were my doctor's words as I sat in her office, nine months pregnant and weighing 187 pounds. She hadn't expected me to gain 52 pounds during my pregnancy. I am a registered dietitian, and food, nutrition, and diets are my business. But like many first-time moms I regarded pregnancy as a time to relax my eating standards. Almost every night I ate a bowl of delicious rich ice cream. I also snacked much more and found that if I didn't eat often I didn't have quite enough energy. In the beginning, food also helped fight nausea.

I really wasn't worried about my weight. I had always been able to maintain my weight between 130 and 135 pounds, which is fine for my five-foot, eight-inch frame. I figured after the baby was born, I would just get back to exercising and eating right and those excess pounds would melt away.

Three hours after my daughter Sarah was delivered by cesarean section, a food tray was brought to me. It carried coffee, red Jell-O, and chicken broth. These bland foods were supposed to restore my energy without taxing my digestive tract.

I hadn't eaten for more than eleven hours and I was hungry but concerned. I contemplated the caffeine-, sodium-, and sugar-laden concoctions before me. Sure, they were safe for me, but what about when I breastfed Sarah? I realized that the foods I ate might pass into my breast milk and could upset or even harm her.

Because I would be nursing my daughter, my eating habits and occasional dietary indiscretions took on new significance. Should I drink coffee? Was the champagne that my husband and I planned to celebrate with safe? Were the pink-foil-wrapped chocolate cigars to be avoided? Could pesticides travel from the foods I ate into my breast milk? How would fatty or cholesterol-rich food affect Sarah? And what about my plans to lose weight, too?

The hospital staff who were so competent at answering my husband's and my questions about breastfeeding techniques, baths, and diapering weren't well informed about diet. They told me, "Eat what you like. If it bothers the baby, then just avoid that food." But general recommendations weren't enough for the nutritionist in me. I wanted scientific studies to back up any eating decisions I made.

When I got home from the hospital, I looked through the breastfeeding and postpartum sections of my pregnancy books for answers to my nutrition questions. Unfortunately, their advice was just too vague: "Eat a balanced diet and avoid gassy food." There was no specific guideline about how much coffee I could drink or information about the effects a glass of wine might have on the baby.

I was also advised not to worry about weight loss. Breastfeeding mothers are told they will automatically lose weight, even while eating the extra 500 calories a day recommended while nursing. In theory, these 500 calories, plus some taken from the mother's stored body fat, are used to make milk for the baby to thrive on. I knew that this wasn't entirely true. Studies have shown that breastfeeding mothers might not automatically lose weight if they follow this advice. Some mothers may require far fewer calories than the 2,700 per day recommended while nursing.

To answer my nutrition questions, I did my own research. I read all the respected lactation textbooks and talked to the experts in the field. I developed a diet for myself that produced safe and gentle weight loss and kept my daughter Sarah happy, healthy, and in the ninetieth percentile for height and weight.

When Sarah was nineteen months old, I was fortunate enough to have another happy, healthy little girl we named Emily. Once again I needed to lose weight, so I put my eating and nutrition plan into practice, and I was able to nurse my daughter, feel good, lose weight, and stay healthy and energetic.

This book is for all mothers who choose to breastfeed their children, but those of you concerned about the weight you gained during pregnancy will find it particularly helpful. Personally, I started to really worry about the way I looked and the rate I was losing weight about six weeks after Sarah was born. At that point, my daughter was thriving and I was confident about my ability to nurse, but I was still twenty-five pounds over my prepregnancy weight and I had never been so tired in my life.

Not all of you will have reached the six-week postpartum stage. You brand-new moms shouldn't even begin to worry about losing weight until at least six weeks after delivery. You should just focus on taking care of yourself and your new baby. For those veteran moms ready to start losing weight, this book will give you the information you need to plan a sensible, gentle weight-loss program. Always keep in mind that your primary goal is to have a safe and satisfying nursing experience.

Some people say that new mothers shouldn't be forced to worry about losing weight because the challenges a new baby brings are all they should have to cope with. Being a sexy, skinny woman is an additional hassle they don't need. I absolutely agree. This book is not about trying to please someone else or about telling women they must look like models in fashion magazines. A new mother is doing the most important job of her life. She should be proud of herself and not be apologetic about some excess bulge around her middle.

I've said it before and I'll keep saying it: while you are breastfeeding, your primary job is to take care of yourself and your baby. It is not the time to be a supermom. Resist the pressure to jump back into the rhythm of your previous life. You had a baby: whether it is your first or your fifth, take it easy on yourself.

But even if you decide that now is not the time to lose weight, it's still the perfect time to look critically at the food that passes over your family table. If your child hasn't started on solid food yet (and he doesn't need to until four to six months old), he will eventually adopt the same eating patterns you have. If you eat lots of snacks or fried foods, then when your child is older and can make choices of his own, he'll eat the same way. So not only do you affect your own health by examining what you eat, you'll influence your child's health, too.

This book isn't just for mothers who want to lose weight; it's for any breastfeeding mom who wants to eat well. In chapter 1, you'll see why your decision to breastfeed is the right one. In chapters 2, 3, and 4, I'll explain how your body makes milk, how the food you eat affects your milk, and which nutrients are particularly important. In chapter 5, I'll discuss weight loss and how you can lose weight safely while breastfeeding.

In chapter 6, I'll show you a simple meal plan for weight loss that is safe for you and won't compromise your baby's health or your breastfeeding experience. In chapter 7, I'll talk about exercise—why it's important to set realistic goals for yourself and find a physical activity that you like. I'll also address the common reasons moms don't exercise and suggest ways for you to overcome those obstacles.

In chapter 8, I'll debunk some of those old wives' tales about foods like chocolate and cabbage upsetting your baby. I'll also discuss more serious concerns about pesticides, caffeine, nicotine, and alcohol passing into your breast milk and affecting your baby's health. Smart food choices can eliminate or minimize the risk these substances pose.

Mothers who have delivered by cesarean or who have health problems such as diabetes, anemia, or high blood pressure will have unique nutrition questions, which will be handled in chapter 9. In chapter 10, you'll find recipes to simplify your life. They are easy to prepare, made with familiar ingredients, and are nutritious, delicious, and freezable.

When I was a brand-new mom, I had tons of questions about nursing my baby. Sure, I knew about food, but nobody ever told me how to pick out a nursing bra that fit right or what to do if my breasts were engorged. In the final chapters, I've included a question-and-answer section as well as a list of excellent resources on breastfeeding and baby care.

I hope this book will give mothers enough information to make smart decisions about what to eat while they breastfeed, so they can feel good about themselves and their decision to nurse their babies. New mothers need to eat well so they'll have nutritious milk to feed their infants and the energy to care for them. My goal is to guide you to a healthy diet that will help you lose weight naturally and safely while you nourish a happy, healthy new child.

EAT WELL,
LOSE WEIGHT,
WHILE BREASTFEEDING

1

THE RIGHT DECISION

This book is intended to help you eat well, lose weight, and feel good about yourself, but that is not all it can do. I also want to support you in your decision to breastfeed your child so that you have a great nursing experience.

Breastfeeding is absolutely the best way to feed your baby, but American society is not always supportive of it. Before you begin reading about what to eat, I want you to appreciate that the feeding choice you made is a great one. I also want you to know that you are not alone if you have some doubts about the choice you've made. Though breastfeeding is wonderful, it also has some drawbacks.

New mothers often doubt that they can breastfeed, even though it is the way nature meant for babies to be fed. Whatever you do, don't interpret these doubts to mean that you aren't capable of breastfeeding. Even women who have had cesareans or twins or who have medical problems can nurse their children.

Take comfort in knowing that you are not the only mom who is fretful about her ability to breastfeed. Judy Jean Chapman, a nurse at Vanderbilt University, studied what new mothers worry about. She found that when first starting to breastfeed, mothers worried most about sore breasts, providing enough milk to feed their babies, and how frequently their babies nursed.

Of course, the mothers also worried about the well-being of their babies. Fussiness, sleepiness, mixed-up days and nights, rashes, the rate of weight gain, and colds were the most frequently reported concerns. When the mothers were questioned about their own postpartum problems, fatigue topped the list. They also expressed concerns about their older children, returning to work or school, and the extra weight they carried. I think anyone who has a frank discussion with a new nursing mom will hear some or all of these concerns. Of all the mothers I know, I can't think of one who approached breastfeeding with absolute confidence. Of course some women are more at ease right from the start, but for many mothers breastfeeding is a skill that must be learned and practiced before it becomes second nature.

Three Tips for Successful Breastfeeding

1. Put your baby to the breast as soon as possible. This is more about contact and bonding than feeding. Most babies do not feed right away, but the skin-to-skin contact will support breastfeeding and mother-to-baby bonding.
2. Tell the hospital staff you do not want formula given to your baby. Providing just 1 ounce of formula can affect breastfeeding success. Make sure your husband or partner, friends, and family understand how important this is to you and ask for their support, too.
3. Allow ample time to breastfeed at each session and throughout the day. The more you nurse, the more you become relaxed and natural at nursing.

If you're feeling overwhelmed by your worries, talk to a mother who has successfully breastfed her babies. If you don't have a friend you can speak to, call the experienced moms of La Leche League. Their contact information is listed in the Resource section at the back of the book. If you are reading this book before you deliver, you may want to call the La Leche League in advance of your birth so you have a mother you know you can talk to. You may also want to contact a lactation consultant, a woman who has special training in the subject of breastfeeding and who can assist you with almost any problem. Ask your hospital, health care provider, or nurse-midwife about the lactation consultant they use or go to page 213 for information about how to locate a consultant in your area.

IS BREAST REALLY BEST?

No matter how unsure you might be about breastfeeding, you'll be happy to know that breastfeeding is the best way to nourish your baby. It is only in the twenty-first century, with our sophisticated medical technology and research, that we have to spend thousands, if not millions, of dollars on studies to prove what Mother Nature and you already know. Studies repeatedly demonstrate that breastfeeding not only provides the ideal food, it also protects against illness by passing some of your disease-fighting antibodies to your child in your milk. Compared to infants who were never breastfed, the breastfed babies who nursed for three or more months needed fewer doctor visits, saving over $331 in medical care in a single year. Dr. Peter Howie reported in the *British Medical Journal* a study of more than six hundred Scottish mothers and their babies from birth to age two. He found that children who were nursed for at least thirteen weeks had significantly fewer reported instances of vomiting and diarrhea than babies who were fed formula.

The protective effect of breastfeeding lasted even after breast milk stopped being a baby's main food. Babies who were nursed less than thirteen weeks seemed to have the same rate of vomiting and diarrhea as the formula-fed babies (while only vomiting and diarrhea were evaluated in this study, other reports show that breastfeeding protects against bronchitis, food poisoning, even influenza). More recent research has found that breastfeeding impacts sudden infant death syndrome (SIDS). While breastfeeding did not eliminate the risk of SIDS, the rate is lower among breastfed infants. Breastfed babies may have lower blood pressure as they get older, too. Researchers followed formula-fed and breast-fed premature babies from birth to age thirteen and from birth to age sixteen and found that the breastfed infants had lower blood pressure as teenagers. According to a Harvard study, breastfeeding improved how the body used blood sugar. The longer a woman breastfed, the lower her risk of developing type 2 diabetes in middle age. The evidence from these recent studies points out that mothers should be encouraged by their doctors to breastfeed at birth and to continue for at least six months to get the maximum protection against disease for their babies.

Women who must return to work soon after delivery are also encouraged to breastfeed for as long as possible. If a bottle or formula must be introduced, these mothers should use the bottle as a supplement, keeping breast milk as the primary food. Better yet, use expressed breast milk to fill that bottle.

The developmental benefits of breastfeeding are endless. Breast-fed babies are likely to have better teeth and less likely to have "nursing bottle syndrome," which occurs when a child is left with a bottle in his or her mouth (usually while sleeping) and the liquid—be it milk, formula, or juice—pools around tiny developing teeth, creating an ideal environment for cavities to form. A breast-fed baby uses her tongue to suck in a way that protects against misaligned teeth. Babies also use more muscles in their mouths when sucking from the breast and this, too, protects against crooked teeth. In addition, breastfed babies are less likely to suck their thumb because nursing allows them to satisfy their need to suck.

Several studies confirm a connection between breastfeeding and intelligence. In a 2002 *Journal of the American Medical Association* study and an earlier study in the journal *Pediatrics,* researchers found that breastfed infants had higher IQs as adults than adults who had not been breastfed. The breastfed babies also tended to do better in reading comprehension, math tests, and school exams. Infants who had been breastfed for seven to nine months had the greatest increase in IQ.

Another big plus is that you can't tamper with breast milk. Formula must be mixed or at the very least poured into bottles and consumed right away or stored and used within twenty-four hours. At any of these preparation stages, it is possible to contaminate the formula. Breast milk comes out of the breast safe and ready to serve. Formulas that require the addition of water can be over- or underdiluted, while breast milk is created in the perfect concentration.

Breast milk is even tailored to the baby's age and nutritional needs. Breast milk is rich in protein at the beginning of a feeding, while the end of the feeding contains more fat, the nutrient that provides lots of good calories and assuages hunger pangs. Mothers of premature babies produce milk that is richer in protein than the milk of mothers of full-term babies. As the premature baby grows, the composition of the mother's milk changes automatically to meet the baby's needs. Within one month it becomes the same as full-term milk.

Another bonus is that a breastfeeding baby drinks exactly as much or as little milk as she wants, and this is a good thing, because only the baby really knows how much she needs. Mothers and babysitters who see that the baby has drunk only half the bottle may feel compelled to make the baby finish that bottle, even though she doesn't really want it or need it, setting the stage for potential eating or weight problems down the road. Breastfeeding an infant for six months is associated with a lower rate of childhood and early adolescent obesity. Incidence of adult obesity appears to be less in those who were breastfed as infants as well. Interestingly, a 2004 *Pediatric* study found breastfeeding for any amount of time also protected babies against being overweight.

Is Your Baby Getting Enough to Eat?

Some breastfeeding moms worry that since they can't see how much their babies drink, they might not be drinking enough. A newborn who wets six or more diapers every day, has two to five bowel movements, has eight to twelve feedings, looks and acts healthy, and is gaining weight is sure to be getting enough breast milk.

Once you and your baby become a "nursing couple," you will quickly discover some of the secondary benefits of breastfeeding. A baby cradled in his mother's arms and nursing at her breast must be the most secure being on earth. He's comforted by the warm skin-to-skin contact. If he glances upward, his twelve-to-fifteen-inch visual range clearly captures his mom's smile and loving eyes. This experience goes a long way toward providing your child with a sound emotional foundation for life.

Your decision to breastfeed has some purely selfish benefits, too. Because you're breastfeeding, you'll have to sit down and put your feet up throughout the day as you nurse your baby. Very small infants may need to nurse every one to two hours, and a ten-month-old may nurse three to five times a day. While the baby eats you really can't do much else, which means you get a little rest, too.

Breastfeeding can help the family budget, since you won't have to buy expensive cans of formula. In 1985 it cost about $300 per year to feed a baby formula. In 2004 that cost was estimated to be $750 to $1,200.

Breastfeeding appears to offer Mom health benefits, too. If you experienced iron-deficiency anemia while pregnant, breastfeeding may help you conserve iron. Breastfeeding often stops menstruation for six to twelve months after you give birth, which means your body won't be losing the iron lost when menstrual bleeding resumes. This temporary cessation of menstruation also reduces your chance of getting pregnant, but please don't count on breastfeeding as a means of birth control—it isn't reliable. Epidemiological studies have found that women have a lower rate of premenopausal breast cancer if they breastfed their babies.

Breastfeeding also helps your body get back in shape. Because your body is making milk for your child, you'll need extra calories, some of which will come from the fat you stored during pregnancy. Breastfeeding also causes your uterus to contract, and this can help return your tummy to its prepregnancy shape.

SOME CHALLENGES OF BREASTFEEDING

Breastfeeding is not without problems. As I mentioned earlier, you're likely to find it stressful at times. Since you are your child's sole source of food, you won't be able to leave her easily for any extended time. In emergencies, or if you plan ahead, you can express a supply of milk and keep it in the freezer until needed. But when your baby wakes up at 1:00 A.M., 3:00 A.M., and 5:00 A.M., it is you she wants. Sure, many dads help by getting up and bringing baby to Mom, but then they get to go back to sleep. You're on duty.

At social events it's often the mother who provides most of the care. In the beginning, when little babies cry unpredictably, the breast is one of the surefire ways to calm them down. If you aren't completely comfortable breastfeeding in public, this will mean finding quiet, out-of-the-way places to nurse and missing out on some of the activities.

When my daughter was a newborn, my husband and I were taking a course in Boston. I could never breastfeed comfortably among strangers. I found myself spending most of my class time in a corner of the ladies' room that fortunately had a comfortable seat. And I remember taking Sarah on her first airplane ride when she was ten weeks old. The plane was packed with businessmen, there were no empty seats, and the aisle seat I requested was taken. I had no elbow room and spent a good deal of the flight in the airplane's restroom nursing Sarah.

There is another side of breastfeeding that most of us veterans don't like to share with new moms because it may be discouraging. Breastfed babies don't sleep the way bottle-fed babies do. In fact, they might sleep less and wake more often.

The "normal" (if there is such a thing) nighttime sleep cycle for newborns is about four to five hours long, which increases to eight to ten hours by the third or fourth month. In all, the "normal" infant sleeps thirteen to fifteen hours out of every twenty-four; this decreases only slightly by the second birthday.

If you can get your child to sleep those eight to ten hours at night and all at once, then the two of you can get some much-needed sleep. Unfortunately, breastfed babies often don't sleep for such long stretches and they might sleep a little less than babies fed formula. In a study of ninety-seven British infants both breast- and formula-fed, at six weeks breastfed babies slept eighty minutes less per day than formula-fed infants. In a study of South Korean infants that compared the behavior patterns of formula- and breast-fed babies, the breastfed infants fed more frequently and longer but their long bouts of sleeping were shorter in duration than those of their formula-fed counterparts.

I share this information with you to let you know that you are not alone if you worry about your child's sleep patterns. Lack of sleep is a big source of concern to mothers and frequent night waking can be a reason some women stop breastfeeding.

Recent studies offer help for tired breastfeeding moms. Researchers at the University of Illinois assigned twenty-six new breastfeeding parents to either a treatment or control group. The treatment parents were asked to offer a "focal feed" between 10 P.M. and 12 A.M. When or if their baby woke again, instead of feeding, they were instructed to offer comfort techniques such as swaddling, walking, or diapering to lengthen the interval to the next feeding. After three weeks the treatment group slept longer and by eight weeks all of the treatment infants were sleeping through the night, whereas only 23 percent of the control group was sleeping through the night. The infants who slept through the night consumed more milk in the morning, but total milk intake did not differ between the two groups. This may be a technique that suits some families, but all families should be encouraged to practice the techniques they are most comfortable with. Many mothers actually enjoy that 2 A.M. feeding and see it as a time for uninterrupted bonding and only a short-term inconvenience.

If you are feeling tired and worn out, you have good reason. Don't get discouraged. Instead, set your priorities. Take care of yourself and your baby. If you can't keep up with the housework, don't be alarmed. Just handle what you can. You can always do it later. What you can't get back is this precious time with your child.

Well-meaning friends will give you all sorts of advice about getting your child to sleep. They'll tell you to introduce solid food early, let your child cry it out, or wean your child.

Some mothers think if they are doing it "right" they shouldn't be having any problems. Not true—all new moms worry, just don't let it undermine your confidence. Women who lack confidence are more likely to turn to supplemental formula feeding and usually stop breastfeeding soon afterward. New mothers are most vulnerable to quitting nursing immediately postpartum when they are on their own in the first two weeks after delivery. Don't be pressured into doing anything that does not feel right to you. It is important and extremely helpful to have someone you can talk to. Find other breastfeeding moms (call some women from your birthing class), contact the La Leche League, or ask your health care provider for advice on finding a good lactation consultant.

Take comfort in knowing that it is normal for newborns to be wakeful, and normal for mothers to have a hard time adjusting to their babies' schedules. I wasn't able to count on either of my girls sleeping through the night until they were about fifteen months old. This might sound ghastly to you, but it wasn't bad. I got used to it and came to enjoy our quiet time together. After their first birthdays they would usually wake up only once in the night, and that was more for reassurance than anything else. By preschool both Sarah and Emily were champion sleepers. I have a secret theory that infants who wake frequently as babies and are comforted by their moms or dads grow up to be sound sleepers.

NEW MOTHERS NEED SUPPORT

Our culture isn't always supportive of mothering or of breast-feeding. Many women must return to full-time jobs while their babies are young, and they worry whether or not they will be able to combine nursing and work. Or their families may not understand why a mother would choose to breastfeed when she can formula-feed. According to the data from the Ross Mothers Survey (RMS), U.S. breastfeeding rates have reached their highest levels. Breastfeeding rates are up because mothers recognize the health benefits of breastfeeding for their baby.

In the 1930s about 70 percent of babies were breastfed; by 1960, that number plunged to 30 percent. The decline in the 1960s was probably the result of the mass marketing of baby formula. In the 1970s there was a strong countertrend and more mothers returned to nursing. But the late 1980s saw a gradual decline in breastfeeding. A 1990 Ross Survey found that 51.4 percent of all babies were breastfed while in the hospital, down from 58 percent in 1985. The data released from the RMS survey in 2003 showed that over 70 percent of today's mothers initiate breastfeeding while in the hospital and over 33 percent of mothers are still breastfeeding at age six months. The National Immunization Survey (NIS), a public health survey conducted by the Centers for Disease Control and Prevention, asked questions about breastfeeding as well as immunization. The NIS survey found that in 2001 almost two-thirds of children had been breastfed, with 27 percent still breastfeeding at six months and 12 percent at twelve months. In 1992 only 19 percent of babies surveyed by Ross were still breastfed at six months. Though the six-month rate has improved in both surveys, it is still not optimal. The U.S. Department of Health and Human Services Healthy People 2010 goal is to have a 50 percent breastfeeding rate at six months of age. Women who work full-time start breastfeeding at the same rate as all mothers, but by age six months 25 percent of the full-time working moms have stopped breastfeeding. Women who are participants in the Special Supplemental Nutrition Program for Women, Infants and Children (WIC) are less likely to be breastfeeding while in the hospital and as a result have lower rates at six months. Rates for breastfeeding at six months are significantly lower for all women who work out of the home.

Returning to work is an often-cited reason for stopping breast-feeding and, in some cases, for not even starting in the first place. The statistics point out that we need to be more supportive of mothers and children. Mothers need adequate facilities for feeding their children at work, and they need on-site affordable child care.

Your breastfed child is very lucky. In the long run you won't regret any inconvenience, and your child will be happier and healthier because of it. Breastfeeding is likely to be one of the first important decisions you make about your baby's health and upbringing. It's one of the only parenting decisions unanimously recognized as being the right one. Breast truly is best.

2

THEY ARE WHAT YOU EAT

Lactation is the natural continuation of your pregnancy. Look upon pregnancy as an eighteen-month experience. The first nine months are for building the baby, the next nine for breastfeeding her. Of course, many mothers breastfeed for longer than nine months. However long you choose to nurse, it's important that you remember to take just as good care of yourself after you have the baby as you did while you were pregnant.

Good care includes good eating. The nutrients you stored and those you eat every day will be what nourishes your baby. At no other time in your life will there be such a demand on your physical resources. If this sounds intimidating, don't fret; your menu does not need to be perfect. Your only job is to provide your body with nutritious food. It will then efficiently and elegantly transform that food into a perfectly balanced blend of nutrients for your baby. While diet plays as big a role in lactation as it does in pregnancy, your day-to-day food choices have little impact on the composition or quantity of your breast milk. Probably the most important thing for you to do is to make the time to eat; too many mothers do not do this. Allow yourself to sit down and eat good food every few hours and you will automatically be nourishing yourself and your baby.

HOW THE BREAST MAKES MILK

During your pregnancy, you no doubt noticed changes in your breasts; they got larger, became tender, and the nipples and areolae (the area around the nipples) darkened. These temporary changes occur in preparation for breastfeeding.

The milk sacs, or alveoli, in your breasts are stimulated by the hormones your body creates during pregnancy. By the second trimester these alveoli can produce early milk, which could help feed a baby born prematurely. Within twenty-four hours of birth, the hormones in your body change again, this time signaling full-scale milk production to begin. These physical and hormonal changes, combined with the stimulation provided by the baby's sucking at the breast, will allow for steady and regular milk production.

The yellow colostrum is the first milk your breasts make. It is extremely rich in protein and carries important disease-fighting antibodies essential to a newborn's health. Colostrum is replaced by true milk a couple of days after delivery. As long as the baby is allowed to feed regularly at the breast, your body will automatically produce an adequate supply of milk, even if you are nursing twins or triplets.

Your breasts increase in size during the time you breastfeed because of the extra blood flowing through them. The blood carries nutrients from your digestive tract to the breast and eventually to your baby. Prepregnancy breast size has nothing to do with a woman's ability to nurse successfully. All women have the same milk-producing equipment. Women with large breasts simply have more fat tissue surrounding the milk-making apparatus.

WHO WILL SUFFER IF MOM'S DIET ISN'T NUTRITIOUS?

The good news is that even if your diet is less than ideal, your body is still able to manufacture nourishing milk. This is Mother Nature's way of ensuring that your baby is well fed. In most cases a mother would have to eat an extremely restricted diet for a long time to create a nutritional deficiency in her breast milk. This can happen, but fortunately it's rare.

However, a diet inadequate in calories and nutrients will have some negative effects. Mothers who can't or won't eat enough good, healthy food are more likely to feel tired and irritable. When combined with the fatigue from caring for a new baby, this adds up to a less than ideal nursing situation. Since fatigue is one of the main reasons women stop nursing, it's vital to eat well to keep your stamina up.

HOW DO YOU KNOW IF YOUR BABY IS EATING ENOUGH?

A newborn baby who feeds about ten times a day at the breast and wets six or more diapers every day is probably getting plenty to eat. Weight checks conducted by your health care provider will also be a good guide. Your child will be weighed and measured at the two-week, two-month, and four-month doctor's visit. Checking weight at home is not recommended because it puts too much emphasis on the scale, and home scales are often inaccurate. Instead, pay attention to your baby's moods. If he appears bright, alert, and happy most of the time, then chances are very good that he is healthy and eating enough.

If you are worried about how often your baby nurses, you aren't alone. Listen to a group of new mothers and you are sure to hear them talk about their feeding worries such as how often baby feeds, falls asleep at the breast, fusses, or even refuses to eat. Do these concerns sound familiar? Don't suffer silently. Talk to your pediatrician or her staff, talk to another mother who is breastfeeding, or call the La Leche League. Support during the first few weeks is important to new moms, so seek it out. When Sarah was six weeks old, we joined a mothers' group of five mothers. A mothers' group is one of the few places you can talk about babies, babies, and babies and not bore everyone to death. Hearing about their problems can help reassure you that you are not alone.

Many mothers comment that their breast milk looks too thin and watery; they worry that it isn't rich enough to nourish their babies. This isn't true. Breast milk is the ideal food for newborns. It may appear thin compared to cow's milk, but it is loaded with the nutrients your baby needs.

It's very hard for new mothers to breastfeed when other family members are not supportive. Older family members may make comments like "You're starving that baby by giving him just breast milk—give him formula or cereal, too." If this happens to you, look for outside support. Try to find another experienced mom who can give you advice and comfort, or contact the La Leche League.

Try not to worry about starting solid foods for the first few months. Most doctors currently recommend that mothers not introduce solid foods to their babies for at least four months. What most of us forget is that breast milk is food—it's just in liquid form. It's perfectly balanced in protein and all the other nutrients that your baby needs.

SHOULD I TAKE A MULTIVITAMIN?

Breastfeeding moms are encouraged to get their nutrition from food, not supplements. Food is simply the most reliable and direct way to get the nutrients you need. A proper diet makes supplements redundant. An orange doesn't contain just vitamin C. It has health-promoting fiber and is a delicious form of energy-providing carbohydrate. A vitamin C tablet contains only vitamin C, with some sort of filler and no energy or fiber. It's not uncommon for mothers to continue prenatal vitamins while they nurse. This is fine, but don't expect a vitamin tablet to replace good, healthy food.

Some breastfeeding mothers, however, really do need to take supplements. A breastfeeding mother who is getting 1,800 calories a day or less will need a balanced multivitamin-mineral supplement because the volume of food she is eating is just too low to meet her nutritional needs. Mothers who are vegetarian and avoid all the animal foods that carry vitamin B_{12} will need to take a B_{12} supplement (2.6 micrograms per day). If a mother isn't eating milk, cheese, or other calcium-rich dairy products, she'll need a calcium supplement. Mothers who avoid vitamin D–fortified food such as milk or cereal and have little exposure to sunlight may be in need of a vitamin D supplement. All these mothers should seek out advice from a physician or nutrition counselor.

HOW DO I CHOOSE A SUPPLEMENT?

Supplements available by prescription and designed for new mothers are good and reliable but are often more expensive than an equally good over-the-counter multivitamin. When selecting a supplement to "round out" your menu, look for one that contains both vitamins and minerals. Read the label. It will contain a list of nutrients included and the percentage of the recommended dietary allowances (RDAs) that they provide. A good supplement to choose while breastfeeding is one that contains most of the nutrients on page 24 along with B vitamins, vitamin D, vitamin E, folic acid, 75 milligrams of vitamin C, some vitamin K, chromium, copper, and selenium. Most multivitamins carry only a small amount of calcium because the full amount can't fit into one pill. Supplements should not exceed the recommended levels based on the RDAs; when taken in excessive amounts, some nutrients can interfere with the absorption of others. See page 20 for the upper limit (UL) for several nutrients.

ARE THERE ANY NUTRIENTS I SHOULD BE CAREFUL ABOUT WHILE NURSING?

There are a few nutrients that, if taken in doses that greatly exceed the RDA, could reach an undesirable level in breast milk. These include vitamin B_6, vitamin D, iodine, and selenium. An excessive dose is more likely to occur when taken as a single nutrient, not as part of a balanced multivitamin.

WILL A MULTIVITAMIN BOOST THE NUTRITIONAL CONTENT OF MY BREAST MILK?

The notion of increasing the nutrients in your milk by taking a multivitamin might have a certain appeal and might even sound logical. Unfortunately, it won't work.

Mothers who are already well nourished won't increase the nutritional quality of their milk by taking multivitamins. Dr. M. Rita Thomas, a researcher specializing in the nutrition needs of breastfeeding mothers, studied the effect supplements would have on well-nourished women who had been nursing for six months. She specifically examined the quantities of vitamin C, vitamin B_6, vitamin B_{12}, folic acid, riboflavin, and thiamine found in their breast milk. She found that the vitamin supplement did not affect the nutrient composition of the breast milk. Please notice that the women studied were already well nourished. Women who have diets that are only marginally adequate and are undernourished themselves can increase the nutritional quality of breast milk by taking supplements.

What you eat while breastfeeding matters. The mother who takes time to eat well will be doing herself and her baby a favor. Don't rely on vitamin and mineral pills alone to provide you with nourishment. Eat health-promoting foods like fruits and vegetables, low-fat protein sources, whole grains, and dairy and your body will be perfectly prepared to make milk your child will thrive upon.

Tolerable Upper Intake Levels for Some Nutrients While Breastfeeding

Tolerable upper intake levels (UL) have been established by the Food and Nutrition Board of the Institute of Medicine. The tolerable UL is the highest daily intake of a nutrient that is not likely to pose a health risk. The UL represents total intake from food, drinks, and supplements. Some supplements will be measured in International Units (IU) or retinol equivalents (RE) and not the milligrams (mg) or micrograms (mcg) used to define the UL. Compare measurements accurately and to be safe, avoid exceeding 100 percent of the RDA as listed on the label.

Vitamin A	1,800–2,000 mg
Vitamin D	50 mcg
Vitamin E	1,800–2,000 mg
Vitamin C	1,800–2,000 mg
Niacin	30–35 mg
Vitamin B_6	80–100 mg
Folate	800–1,000 mg
Choline	3.0–3.5 g
Boron	17–20 mg*
Calcium	2.5 g
Copper	8,000–10,000 mcg
Fluoride	10 mg
Iodine	900–1,100 mcg
Iron	45 mg

Magnesium	350 mg
Manganese	9–11 mg
Molybdenum	1,700–2,000 mcg
Nickel	1.0 mg
Phosphorous	4 g
Selenium	400 mcg
Zinc	34–40 mg
Sodium	2.3 g

*Boron—potentially dangerous; avoid during pregnancy and lactation.

3

WHAT EVERY MOTHER NEEDS
TO KNOW ABOUT NUTRITION
WHILE BREASTFEEDING

This chapter is about helping mothers make smart choices. Gross nutritional deficiencies are unlikely for most nursing mothers in America, but subtle nutrient inadequacies may be a problem. I know from talking to many clients that not everyone is sitting down to three balanced meals a day. I also know that new mothers have a hard time trying to feed themselves and keep up with all their other commitments. The good news is that women who eat conventional diets that include a wide variety of foods are extremely unlikely to have serious nutrition problems. Most nutrients are not difficult to get if smart food choices are made. Even if a mother falls a bit short of meeting the recommended allowances set by the National Academy of Sciences, there is likely to be little impact on her breast milk.

For years the nutritional recommendations for nursing mothers has been quite general: "Eat a little more of all the food groups and you'll do fine." This is not bad advice; it's just not very specific. Some mothers need to learn more about nutrition and change their diets so that they get enough of the foods they really do need. For instance, the levels of selenium and iodine in your breast milk are dependent on how much of these nutrients you eat. If you take supplements, large doses of nutrients such as vitamin B_6, vitamin D, iodine, and selenium might increase the levels of these nutrients in your breast milk to a point that could be detrimental to your baby.

While you are nursing, your need for calcium, magnesium, zinc, folic acid, and vitamin B_6 goes up dramatically, and it's important to select foods rich in these nutrients. It is particularly vital for you to pay attention to the amount of calcium and folic acid you consume, since these nutrients will be kept constant in breast milk at your expense. It is not yet known for sure, but mothers who don't get enough calcium while nursing may be at greater risk for developing osteoporosis when they get older.

Recognizable deficiencies of thiamine, vitamin B_6, biotin, vitamin B_{12}, and vitamins D and K have been found in breastfeeding mothers who weren't eating enough of the foods they needed. These deficiencies have occurred in mothers in third-world countries where food was simply not available. When deficiencies in babies as well as mothers have occurred in the United States, they have been the result of extremely rigid, restricted diets that mostly consisted of vegetables. Some of the more dramatic cases in this country have occurred with vitamin D and vitamin B_{12} deficiencies. This may sound alarming, but in truth a mother will not be able to create a nutritional deficiency in her baby unless her diet is extremely limited.

Nutritional requirements are different for women of childbearing age and for pregnant and lactating women (see table 1). Some requirements for breastfeeding women, such as that for protein, can be easily met, while other requirements, such as those for zinc, iron, and calcium, are often inadequate in the diet of new mothers. Breastfeeding creates unique demands on your body, and a few nutrients are particularly critical while you're nursing (see table 2). These nutrients are either hard to get, extremely important to mother or baby, or potentially harmful if taken in excessive amounts.

Table 1. Just What a Woman Needs

These recommendations assume a woman is in good health and moderately active. Adolescents may have greater nutritional needs, since they may still be growing during pregnancy and lactation.

Nutrient	Nonpregnant 19–50	Pregnant ≤18	Pregnant 19–50	Lactating ≤18	Lactating 19–50
Protein	46 g	71 g	71 g	71 g	71 g
Vitamin A	700 mcg	750 mcg	770 mcg	1,200 mcg	1,300 mcg
Vitamin D	5 mcg	5 mcg	5 mcg	5 mcg	5 mcg
Vitamin E	15 mg	15 mg	15 mg	15 mg	15 mg
Vitamin K	90 mcg	75 mcg	90 mcg	75 mcg	90 mcg
Vitamin C	75 mg	80 mg	85 mg	115 mg	120 mg
Thiamine	1.1 mg	1.4 mg	1.4 mg	1.4 mg	1.4 mg
Riboflavin	1.1 mg	1.4 mg	1.4 mg	1.6 mg	1.6 mg
Niacin	14 mg	18 mg	18 mg	17 mg	17 mg
Vitamin B_6	1.3 mg	1.9 mg	1.9 mg	2.0 mg	2.0 mg
Folic acid	400 mcg	600 mcg	600 mcg	500 mcg	500 mcg
Vitamin B_{12}	2.4 mcg	2.6 mcg	2.6 mcg	2.8 mcg	2.8 mcg
Calcium	1,000 mg	1,300 mg	1,000 mg	1,300 mg	1,000 mg
Phosphorus	700 mg	1,250 mg	700 mg	1,250 mg	700 mg
Magnesium	310 mg	400 mg	350 mg	360 mg	310 mg
Iron	18 mg	27 mg	27 mg	10 mg	9 mg
Zinc	8 mg	13 mg	11 mg	14 mg	12 mg
Iodine	150 mcg	220 mcg	220 mcg	290 mcg	290 mcg
Selenium	55 mcg	60 mcg	60 mcg	70 mcg	70 mcg
Potassium	4,700 mg	4,700 mg	4,700 mg	5,100 mg	5,100 mg

Some of these numbers might vary from those you see on labels. Labels carry the U.S. RDA. These are numbers for healthy adult men and women. While breastfeeding, the RDA for all nutrients increases, hence the variation. Notice, too, that vitamin A and vitamin E are no longer measured in international units (IU). The new measurements, which are thought to be more accurate, are in mcg (retinol activity equivalents) for vitamin A and mg for vitamin E.

Most of a woman's nutrient requirements increase steadily with the demands of pregnancy and early lactation. By the second six months of lactation, a baby is getting more of his nourishment from solid foods and less from breast milk, which decreases the nutrients needed by his mother.

Table 2. Critical Nutrients for Breastfeeding Women

Nutrients That Are Very Important to Obtain in Food

Calcium	Vitamin B_6
Zinc	Folic acid
Magnesium	

Nutrients Difficult to Obtain on Low-Calorie or Restricted Diets

Calcium	Iron
Zinc	Vitamin E
Magnesium	Riboflavin
Vitamin B_6	Selenium (possibly)
Folic acid	Niacin (possibly)
Thiamine	

Nutrients Easily Obtained from Conventional Diets

Protein	Vitamin A
Fat	Vitamin D
Sodium	Vitamin K
Potassium	Vitamin B_{12}
Copper	Biotin
Vitamin C	Iodine
Pantothenic acid	Manganese
Fluoride	Chromium
Molybdenum	

Nutrients That Might Be Harmful if Overconsumed as Supplements

Vitamin B_6	Iodine
Vitamin D	Selenium

VITAL NUTRIENTS FOR THE
BREASTFEEDING MOTHER

To help you evaluate your diet and plan healthy menus, I'll discuss every major nutrient on the following pages, explaining the
role each plays in promoting good health. Keep in mind that nutrients have the same health-promoting effect for your baby as
they do for you. The recommendations given here are based on
the U.S. Dietary Reference Intakes (DRIs) established for breastfeeding mothers.

Protein

Protein is your body's basic building material. Muscles, organs,
bones, cartilage, skin, antibodies, enzymes, and some hormones
are all made from protein. You need it and so does your baby. Each
day, a nursing mother secretes about 6 to 11 grams of protein in
her breast milk to nourish her baby. A breastfeeding mother needs
an extra 25 grams of protein each day to meet the protein needs of
her and her baby. One extra glass of milk, along with 2 to 3 ounces
of extra chicken, fish, or meat at meals can meet this demand.

In most cases, getting adequate protein is not difficult, provided you eat foods like eggs, beef, chicken, and milk. In a study
of middle-class American breastfeeding mothers, it was found
that these women ate, on average, 94 grams of protein a day, significantly more than the recommended protein intake. Vegetarians need to pay more attention to their protein intake, but they
can easily get enough of this nutrient by making intelligent food
choices (read about the vegetarian diet in chapter 9). A glass of
milk provides 8 grams of protein, one egg contains 7 grams, and
a cup of cooked beans will provide a mother with 13 grams.

We can't store protein as we do some other nutrients, so we
need a new supply every day. Protein deficiency is most likely to
become a problem when budgets get tight. Protein-rich foods like
beef, chicken, and fish are expensive. If a mother isn't able to eat
the recommended amount of protein, the protein for her baby

will be drawn from the mother's muscle tissue, sapping the mother's strength and even increasing her chances for illness. Poor nutrition will have little impact on the protein content of breast milk, whereas eating extra protein might increase overall milk volume but not the protein content of milk.

Many of the protein-rich foods I've listed contain other vital nutrients, such as zinc and iron. Unfortunately, protein-rich animal foods also contain cholesterol and saturated fats. You can reduce the fat by trimming your meats, removing the skin from poultry, and choosing low-fat dairy products.

Some experts believe that eating too much protein interferes with the body's calcium balance, thus increasing our risk of osteoporosis as we get older. Excessive intake of protein may also be connected with kidney disease in old age, perhaps because the kidneys become overworked from trying to eliminate excessive by-products of protein digestion.

Protein is very important for nursing mothers, but don't overdo it. You can get too much of a good thing. A nursing mother needs at least two good protein sources daily, such as meat, fish, chicken, or protein alternative (dairy, beans, peanut butter, tofu, veggie burgers, nuts). The small but significant protein in bread, rice, and cereal add up to be the second greatest source of protein in a woman's diet.

Good sources of protein: chicken, beef, fish, turkey, cheese, eggs, milk, yogurt, grains (oatmeal, brown rice, pasta, whole wheat bread), and legumes and nuts (peanuts, cashews, almonds, lentils, soybeans, kidney beans, tofu).

Even if you don't eat much meat, a small amount of animal protein such as a few ounces of hamburger or ground turkey scrambled into a spaghetti sauce significantly boosts the protein value of a meal.

Vitamin A

Vitamin A does much more than promote good vision. It keeps skin healthy, helps make some essential hormones, assists the immune system, and even helps make red blood cells.

A healthy American mother passes about 400 to 670 micrograms of vitamin A each day to her baby through her breast milk. A nursing mom must consume an extra 500 to 600 micrograms of vitamin A each day, for a total of 1,200 micrograms daily. The mother's need for vitamin A drops a bit in the second six months of nursing, to 1,200 micrograms, since the baby starts to get more nutrients from solid foods.

Women in wealthy industrialized nations like the United States are unlikely to be vitamin A deficient or produce vitamin-deficient milk. Mother Nature recognizes the importance of vitamin A and arms the female body with enough storage capacity to prevent deficiencies. Well-nourished mothers usually have about 200 milligrams of vitamin A stored in their bodies. A baby who breastfeeds exclusively for the first six months and then partially until the first birthday will consume about 192 milligrams of vitamin A. Even if a mother didn't eat any food containing vitamin A (which would be extremely difficult, if not impossible, to do), her breastfeeding baby would still not entirely deplete his mother's stores of vitamin A.

Vitamin A is fat soluble, which means the body stores any excess in fat tissue. Toxic reactions can occur if supplements are used at amounts that far exceed the DRI. These toxic reactions can include headache, vomiting, and liver damage. Mothers who take extremely large doses of vitamin A run the risk of increasing the vitamin A content of their breast milk to an unhealthy level. The UL for vitamin A is 2,800 micrograms.

Good sources of vitamin A: liver, eggs, milk, sweet potato, carrot, spinach, winter squash, greens, cantaloupe, mango, papaya, tomato, and apricot.

Deep orange, green, or red foods are usually very good sources of vitamin A, as are most fruits and vegetables. Studies have found that the vitamin A content of breast milk actually increases in spring and summer when we eat more vitamin A–rich produce.

Vitamin D

Vitamin D works with calcium and phosphorus to harden or mineralize your and your baby's bones. Vitamin D deficiency can cause rickets, a disorder in which bones don't form properly. In parts of the world where people don't or can't consume enough vitamin D, children develop rickety bowed legs when they start to walk. Their soft bones are so weak that they bow under the child's weight. Fortunately, rickets is quite rare in the United States.

We can get our vitamin D from food and supplements, or our bodies can manufacture it when we're exposed to sunlight. The DRI for vitamin D for a pregnant and nursing mother is 5 micrograms, the same amount required by a nonpregnant woman under age fifty. A baby will consume only about 0.3 to 0.6 micrograms in a full day's supply of breast milk. Vitamin D deficiency risk increases in premature infants and women who do not drink vitamin D–fortified milk. A glass of vitamin D–fortified milk carries 100 IU per quart or 2.5 micrograms. Much of vitamin D works with calcium to maintain the mother's good health.

Vitamin D deficiencies have only been found in breastfed babies born to mothers who ate diets completely lacking vitamin D and who also limited their babies' exposure to sunlight. Sunlight converts vitamin D precursors in the body into the real thing. Your baby can get a week's supply of vitamin D by spending two hours outside without a hat or thirty minutes in the sun wearing just a diaper. Babies with dark skin may need slightly longer exposure. To protect skin, dermatologists recommend limiting sun exposure and wearing sunscreen. Acknowledging adequate sun exposure can be difficult to determine, the American Academy of Pediatrics and the Centers for Disease Control (CDC) have recommended that all exclusively breastfed babies be supplemented with vitamin D beginning at two months of age. Check with your child's pediatrician before starting your baby on a supplement.

Don't start self-prescribing large quantities of vitamin D for you or your baby. If you take too much of this vitamin, potentially toxic amounts can be secreted into your breast milk. Supplements that exceed the DRI levels are not advised; the UL for vitamin D is 50 micrograms.

Good sources of vitamin D: vitamin D–fortified milk (one cup supplies about 25 percent of the vitamin D needed by adults), vitamin D–fortified margarine, eggs, liver, and fish. There are no reliable plant sources of this nutrient.

Vitamin E

Vitamin E helps protect the muscles, cardiovascular system, and nerve membranes from the damaging reactions that are a normal part of metabolism. It also helps the body use vitamin A. Vitamin E deficiency can show up as a certain type of anemia or as a degeneration and weakness of the muscles, but it is rare unless an individual cannot absorb fat properly.

The DRI for vitamin E is set higher than the amount you'll actually need because your body may not efficiently absorb this nutrient from food. Your baby will be taking in 1.4 to 2.3 milligrams of vitamin E in the breast milk he drinks every day. To meet your own needs for vitamin E and the needs of your nursing baby, the DRI is set at 15 milligrams. Colostrum, the first milk your baby drinks, is extremely rich in vitamin E. In the first days of life, your baby will more than triple his own blood levels of this nutrient.

Your own vitamin E intake may not meet the DRI unless you select food wisely and eat enough calories. It has been estimated that a mother eating only 1,800 calories may ingest only 9 milligrams of vitamin E daily.

One study reports that a mother consuming 27 milligrams per day of vitamin E increased the vitamin E concentration in her breast milk to 11 milligrams per liter (the usual concentration is 2.3 milligrams per liter). Large doses of vitamin E while breast-feeding are not recommended.

Good sources of vitamin E: plant oils (corn oil, vegetable oil, margarine), salad dressing, wheat germ, butter, liver, egg yolk, nuts, seeds, and green leafy vegetables.

Vitamin K

Vitamin K is called the blood-clotting nutrient in honor of its most important function. Vitamin K is so abundant in food that adult women get much more than they actually need. The DRI is set at 90 micrograms daily for women age nineteen and above; only 1.3 to 2.1 micrograms are secreted into breast milk. Even though a mother may eat adequate amounts of this nutrient, breast milk is naturally low in vitamin K. A liter of breast milk contains only 2 micrograms, while an equal amount of formula fortified with vitamin K contains over 20 micrograms. No toxicity from formula has been reported.

All babies have to develop the ability to clot blood, which makes them immediately dependent on an external source of vitamin K. Even thriving newborns can develop a hemorrhaging syndrome caused by vitamin K deficiency. To prevent this potentially lethal condition, the American Academy of Pediatrics recommends that all newborns get a onetime injection of vitamin K, which is administered soon after birth and takes care of the hemorrhaging risk.

Well-nourished mothers who eat good foods like green leafy vegetables and have adequate stores of vitamin K won't increase the vitamin K content of their breast milk, even if they consume extra vitamin K foods or supplements.

Good sources of vitamin K: green leafy vegetables, Brussels sprouts, cabbage, milk, meat, eggs, cereal, fruit, and liver.

Vitamin C

Vitamin C helps form collagen, the substance that supports bones and teeth. It is an antioxidant, which means it protects other vital substances in the body from harmful chemical reactions. It also helps fight infection and assists with the absorption of iron.

While you're pregnant, the vitamin C concentration of your blood actually decreases. This probably occurs because your blood volume increases and your blood becomes more dilute. Your baby, on the other hand, has a vitamin C concentration in his blood twice that of yours.

The vitamin C content of breast milk can vary a bit depending on how many vitamin C–rich foods are eaten daily. Your baby consumes 24 to 40 milligrams of this important nutrient each day from your breast milk. You'll need to eat 115 to 120 milligrams of vitamin C daily to meet the needs of you and your baby.

Getting enough vitamin C for both of you is not hard to do, provided you make fruits, vegetables, or juices part of meals. If your intake of vitamin C is poor, breast-milk concentration will be maintained with vitamin C from your own body reserves. However, since body stores of vitamin C are minimal, you can't rely on them to meet your needs. Instead, make sure to eat vitamin C foods daily.

Recognizable vitamin C deficiency is rare today, but reports in older literature document a case of scurvy in a breastfed baby whose mother wasn't consuming enough vitamin C. The concentration of vitamin C in breast milk goes up a bit during the summer, when more fruits and vegetables are eaten. Supplements can increase concentrations of this nutrient in breast milk if the mother's diet has been deficient. Studies show that the vitamin C content of breast milk will level off at 50 to 60 milligrams per liter if a mother's intake meets or exceeds 100 milligrams daily.

Good sources of vitamin C: citrus fruits (oranges, grapefruits, tangerines, and so on), juices made from these fruits, fortified fruit juices, and most vegetables (dark green leafy vegetables, tomatoes, even potatoes and peppers).

Keep in mind that a real plus of getting enough vitamin C is that it enhances iron absorption. This is critical to your baby—and to you, too, since many moms have low iron stores during pregnancy and lactation.

Thiamine (Vitamin B₁)
Thiamine is a member of the B vitamin family. It helps in energy production and the maintenance of a normal appetite and ner-

vous system. Your need for thiamine increases from 1.1 milligrams when not nursing to 1.4 milligrams while you're breastfeeding. Only about 0.13 to 0.21 milligram of that will be consumed by your baby via breast milk. The thiamine requirement for a nursing mother is set quite a bit higher than what her baby consumes because thiamine plays a vital role in turning all the extra food and energy a mother consumes into breast milk.

Thiamine is not a hard nutrient to obtain, but wise food selections must be made. It is estimated by the National Academy of Sciences, Subcommittee on Nutrition During Lactation that a mother eating between 1,800 and 2,200 calories a day will fall short of the recommended amount of thiamine. Fortunately, the DRI has a safety margin, and even though your thiamine intake might be a bit below the DRI, vitamin deficiency won't occur unless your diet is missing this nutrient for a very long time.

Low intakes of thiamine by mothers can result in lower thiamine concentrations in breast milk. In countries where mothers consume most of their calories from white rice that is not fortified with thiamine, breastfed babies have developed infantile beriberi, the disease caused by thiamine deficiency.

Good sources of thiamine: enriched bread or cereal; whole grain bread, cereal, and pasta; beans, nuts, meat, and liver.

Riboflavin
Riboflavin is another B vitamin. Like thiamine, it plays a role in energy production. It also promotes good vision and healthy skin.

Your baby will consume 0.21 to 0.35 milligram of riboflavin every day from your breast milk. To replace that and meet your own needs, the DRI is set at 1.6 milligrams. The DRI is set quite a bit higher than the amount the baby needs because mothers don't utilize riboflavin with 100 percent efficiency. The riboflavin content of breast milk seems to decline naturally with prolonged breastfeeding. This reflects the baby's need to start on solid foods himself so he can meet his own riboflavin needs.

Though there are no reported cases of riboflavin deficiencies in exclusively breastfed babies, mothers on low-calorie diets of 1,800 calories or less are at risk of not meeting their full DRI. Studies show that riboflavin supplements can increase the content of this nutrient in breast milk even in mothers who eat an adequate diet. I have not come across any reports of excessive intakes or toxicity caused by riboflavin supplements, but it's still wise not to go overboard.

Good sources of riboflavin: milk, yogurt, cheese, whole grains, enriched bread and cereal, and green leafy vegetables.

Niacin

This water-soluble vitamin is found in food, but it can also be made in your body from the amino acid tryptophan. Niacin plays an integral role in our use and transfer of energy. It helps in the metabolism of sugar, fat, and alcohol and even works to keep our skin healthy.

While you were pregnant, your body became better at converting tryptophan to niacin, thereby guaranteeing adequate supplies. A breastfeeding mom will secrete 0.9 to 1.5 milligrams of niacin in her milk each day. Milk from a well-nourished mother is adequate to meet her baby's needs. The DRI for nursing mothers is set at 17 milligrams of niacin. Even on a diet of only 1,800 calories a day, this level can be met if smart food choices are made. If for some reason you aren't able to eat enough niacin-rich foods, your body will convert tryptophan into niacin to meet your needs.

The niacin content of breast milk is directly affected by the food you eat, and niacin supplements can increase milk concentration. So choose supplements wisely.

Good sources of niacin: all protein foods (eggs, meat, poultry, fish, turkey, and tuna), whole wheat bread, enriched pasta, cereal, bread, and nuts.

Vitamin B_6

Vitamin B_6 is extremely important for breastfeeding mothers, and it is the nutrient most likely to be low in breast milk if the mom's diet is inadequate. It assists in the proper metabolism of protein and fats and in the conversion of tryptophan to niacin. It also helps to make red blood cells.

Many mothers don't eat enough foods rich in vitamin B_6. You need 2.0 milligrams of this nutrient each day while breastfeeding; 0.06 to 0.09 milligram will be secreted in your breast milk. Many women eating low-calorie diets consume only 1.4 milligrams of vitamin B_6 daily. Don't take mega doses of vitamin B_6. Doses in the 300- to 600-milligram range have been observed to decrease milk production. Large doses of vitamin B_6 have been shown to cause neurological damage in women taking this nutrient for premenstrual syndrome. Select supplements cautiously if you use them. Doses of 2 to 6 milligrams do not appear to suppress milk production or cause dangerous side effects, but the National Academy of Sciences, Subcommittee on Nutrition During Lactation does not recommend the routine use of vitamin B_6 supplements for breastfeeding moms. It's best to meet your needs by selecting foods rich in vitamin B_6.

Good sources of vitamin B_6: meats, shellfish, chicken, turkey, eggs, beans, bananas, cauliflower, potatoes, whole grains, soybeans, and sunflower seeds.

Folic Acid

Folic acid, also known as folate and folacin, helps form hemoglobin in red blood cells and build new cells. Folic acid is frequently supplemented during pregnancy because it can prevent neural tube defects. During pregnancy your folic acid requirement is set at 600 micrograms. For breastfeeding moms, the requirement drops to 500 micrograms. A day's supply of breast milk will contain about 50 to 83 micrograms of folic acid. (Human breast milk is a very good source of folic acid when compared to the milk of other animals. Goat's milk has only 10 micrograms per liter; half of the folic acid in cow's milk is destroyed when boiled or prepared for evaporated milk.)

Only about half of the folic acid you ingest gets absorbed, but the DRI is set high enough to allow for this inefficiency. A mother won't have much folic acid stored in her body because most excess folic acid is excreted in the urine. A mother can store about 6 milligrams of folic acid in her body, but after six months of exclusively breastfeeding, 12 milligrams will have been used. Simple math shows that a mother's reserves will be depleted unless she eats foods rich in folic acid. Foods must be selected carefully on a low-calorie diet: the average mother eating 1,800 calories per day will ingest only 261 micrograms, while a mother eating 2,200 calories will consume about 319 micrograms.

Multivitamins and fortified cereals can enhance the folic acid content of the menu and the folic acid content of the breast milk of women deficient in this nutrient. Women with the folic acid deficiency called megaloblastic anemia will find that any dietary folic acid will go first to her breast milk to prevent the same anemia in her child.

Good sources of folic acid: green leafy vegetables, beans, seeds, liver, eggs, and wheat germ, fortified breakfast cereals, and other grain foods.

Vitamin B_{12}

Vitamin B_{12} is a critical nutrient. It works with folic acid to build healthy red blood cells, and it also makes up part of the covering around nerve fibers. Vitamin B_{12} deficiency shows up as a creeping paralysis or a blood anemia characterized by large, immature red blood cells.

The DRI of vitamin B_{12} while you are breastfeeding is set at 2.8 micrograms; you'll be happy to know that this isn't hard to meet. It is estimated that even on as little as 1,800 calories a day, a mother will be able to ingest 5.2 micrograms. At 2,700 calories a day, that jumps to 7.8 micrograms.

It is thought that an infant needs about 0.4 to 0.5 microgram daily, and studies show that mothers eating a good diet will secrete 0.6 to 1.0 microgram each day in their breast milk. To reduce the risk of B_{12} deficiency even more, Mother Nature gives newborns a supply of vitamin B_{12} that can last as long as eight months—if their mothers have consumed enough B_{12} while they were pregnant.

A mother who eats animal foods such as beef, chicken, or dairy products can easily meet her vitamin B_{12} needs. Because fruits and vegetables are practically void of this essential nutrient, mothers who are strict vegetarians are at risk of B_{12} deficiency. A breastfed baby may show signs of the deficiency before his mother does.

To prevent B_{12} deficiency, pregnant and breastfeeding mothers who avoid all animal foods must take foods fortified with vitamin B_{12} or take a 2.6-microgram supplement daily to provide the DRI. (If you are a vegetarian mother, read more about this in chapter 9.)

Good sources of vitamin B_{12}: any food of animal origin (beef, pork, lamb, turkey, chicken, fish, shellfish, milk, yogurt, cheese, and eggs), soy milk, breakfast cereal fortified with B_{12}, and nutritional yeast fortified with B_{12}.

Calcium

Calcium is the predominant mineral in bones and teeth, helping to build them and keep them strong. Calcium also helps muscles and nerves work properly, and it even plays a role in blood clotting and in regulating blood pressure. Deficiency in childhood can show up as stunted bone growth; in adult women, the condition known as osteoporosis (weak, thin bones) has been linked with inadequate calcium intake.

While you are breastfeeding, your DRI is set at 1,000 milligrams daily and 1,300 for women under age eighteen. It can be very difficult, if not impossible, to meet this recommended intake if you aren't eating or drinking dairy products. Women on low-calorie diets (in the 1,800-calorie-per-day range) may be consuming only 715 milligrams, significantly less than the recommended amount.

Because this nutrient is so important, your body has some safety mechanisms that may go into effect if you don't eat enough calcium-rich foods. Studies have shown that women with chronically low calcium intake may be more efficient at utilizing the calcium they do eat. The DRI takes into account that your body is only 40 to 50 percent efficient at turning the calcium you eat as food into the calcium that will go into your breast milk.

At this point, you may be worrying that your calcium intake isn't good enough and your baby isn't getting enough of this vital nutrient. Rest easy. Once again, Mother Nature built a safety mechanism to protect your baby. The calcium content of your breast milk will remain constant, but it will be done at your expense. If you don't eat enough calcium, your body will release calcium from your bones to make up the difference in your breast milk.

Because of this potential for increased calcium drain, there is concern that breastfeeding mothers might have an increased risk of osteoporosis. At this time there's not enough data to say how breastfeeding affects a woman's risk of osteoporosis. Some research suggests that breastfeeding itself may protect women from this disease.

If you are under age twenty-five, make sure you get lots of calcium. At this age, your bones still need to increase their strength by increasing their calcium content.

Black women have diets that average 30 percent lower in calcium than those of white women. Low-income mothers also tend to have diets lower in calcium. Mothers who don't like or can't drink milk need to search out calcium-rich alternatives. (If you don't drink milk, read about what to do in chapter 9.)

Good sources of calcium: milk, cheese, yogurt, fish with edible bones, tofu processed with calcium sulfate, bok choy, broccoli, kale, greens (collard, mustard, and turnip), and bread made with milk.

Phosphorus

Phosphorus is second only to calcium as the mineral in greatest quantity in your body. Most of it is found bound with calcium in bones and teeth. But it also makes up part of phospholipids (a type of fat) and is part of the buffer system that maintains the acid-base balance in your body. Phosphorus must also be present for your body to properly absorb calcium. The good news is that phosphorus is so abundant that deficiency isn't generally a problem.

Calcium and phosphorus are thought to be utilized best if they are present in equal amounts; therefore, the DRI for phosphorus is 700 milligrams for women over age eighteen and 1,250 milligrams for women under age eighteen. The amount of phosphorus in your blood is very tightly regulated so that it stays at a constant level. What you eat, meal to meal, has very little impact on the phosphorus level of your breast milk.

Good sources of phosphorus: animal foods (all meats, fish, poultry, milk, and other dairy products) and soft drinks.

An excessive amount of high-phosphorus food without adequate calcium-containing foods is undesirable and may impact bone health.

Magnesium

Magnesium plays a necessary role in the release of energy. It also assists in proper muscle function and helps to keep calcium in teeth, which in turn helps prevent cavities.

If you eat lots of vegetables and whole grains, your diet is already rich in magnesium. Deficiencies aren't common except in illnesses associated with protracted vomiting or diarrhea, or in kidney disease. Scientists believe that a reservoir of magnesium is kept in our bones to prevent deficiencies.

About 21 to 35 milligrams of magnesium are secreted in breast milk daily, but your DRI is set at 310 to 320 milligrams if you are nineteen or older and 360 milligrams if under age eighteen. The DRI is high because only half of the magnesium you eat is actually absorbed. Many mothers who don't eat vegetables and whole grains may just barely be meeting their magnesium needs.

Breastfeeding mothers consuming fewer than 2,200 calories a day will probably not be getting the recommended level of magnesium. On average, black women consume about 20 percent less magnesium in their diets than white women. This is because they select foods that contain less magnesium. Fortunately, cases of magnesium deficiency in breastfeeding moms are quite rare. Supplements of magnesium do not appear to increase magnesium concentration in breast milk.

Good sources of magnesium: nuts, seeds, legumes, whole grains, green vegetables, scallops, and oysters. Small amounts of magnesium are distributed in many foods, including spinach, tofu, sesame seeds, sunflower seeds, black-eyed peas, garbanzo beans, shrimp, beet greens, broccoli, navy beans, and lima beans.

Iron

Iron is a major part of the blood protein hemoglobin, which carries oxygen throughout your body. Women are particularly at risk for iron deficiencies because we lose iron every month during menstruation. Studies show that as many as 14 percent of women between the ages of fifteen and forty-four may have impaired iron status because of poor diet. During pregnancy menstruation stops, but demands on iron increase: the baby requires iron from you, the placenta also takes iron, and blood is lost during childbirth. Your need for iron is most critical in the second half of your pregnancy.

Breastfeeding itself uses very little iron—only about 0.15 to 0.3 milligram per day. This is less than the amount of iron that would have been lost during menstruation. Since breastfeeding often delays the return of menstruation, your iron stores can have a chance to replenish themselves while you breastfeed if your diet is rich in iron. Since the demand for iron seems less critical while breastfeeding, the DRI is set at 9 milligrams, down from the 27 milligrams you needed while you were pregnant.

If your periods resume while you are still nursing, the demands on your iron reserves can be quite high. You'll have to make sure you eat lots of iron-rich foods. If your intake is poor, you, not your baby, will suffer from anemia.

Iron deficiency in children is a serious problem. In the United States, children between the ages of one and two are at the greatest risk of iron deficiency; they have used up the stores they were born with and now must rely on iron from food sources.

Breastfeeding is a superb way to get iron into your baby. It is estimated that half of the iron in human milk is absorbed by infants, while only 7 percent of the iron in formula is absorbed. It is the lactoferrin, or "milk iron," in breast milk that helps your infant absorb iron and even helps her to fight intestinal infections.

Mothers who only partially breastfeed their babies will want to make sure that the other feedings, whether formula or introductory baby foods, are rich in iron. Infants exclusively breastfed at age seven months were not likely to be anemic at age one and two, but infants breastfed for shorter periods than the seven months had a greater risk of iron deficiency if adequate iron from food was not supplemented.

Your coffee drinking can also affect your baby's iron status. In Costa Rica, mothers drinking more than three cups of coffee a day while pregnant and breastfeeding had lower concentrations of iron in their breast milk, and their babies' iron status was affected by the time they were one month old. (Read more about coffee in chapter 8.) Iron absorption can be enhanced by eating a vitamin C–rich food with every meal. Don't, however, count on milk to help with iron; it is a very poor source of iron.

Good sources of iron: red meat, liver, fish, poultry, shellfish, eggs, beans, dried fruit, oysters, spinach, lima beans, dried peaches, navy beans, soybeans, and kidney beans.

Zinc

Zinc plays many vital roles, helping to maintain the good health of your eyes, liver, kidneys, muscles, skin, and reproductive organs.

The need for zinc is greater during the first six months of breastfeeding than at any other time in a woman's life. The DRI is 12 to 14 milligrams. Meeting this requirement is not easy to do, even for a woman consuming 2,700 calories a day. At lower calorie intakes, mothers may be getting only half to two-thirds of the RDA.

The RDA for zinc for breastfeeding mothers is set quite high, at least four to thirteen times the amount they will pass to their babies in milk (a mother will secrete about 0.9 to 1.5 milligrams of zinc daily in her breast milk in the first six months).

Zinc and Baby Food

Babies need their zinc. Breast milk meets the need for zinc but traditional introductory baby foods such as cereal, fruit, and vegetables have a modest zinc intake. Meat is an excellent source of zinc. Don't be surprised if you hear your health care provider suggesting meat as an early infant food.

The good news is that low intakes by the mother are not generally reflected in a lower zinc concentration in her breast milk. Once again, however, your body may drain your own zinc reserves to provide for your baby if you don't consume enough of this important mineral.

Breast milk is rich in zinc, and colostrum is eight times richer in zinc than mature milk. The zinc found in breast milk is extremely absorbable. The zinc in formula is less so; formula must contain extra zinc to ensure the baby gets enough.

In general, severe zinc deficiencies are not found in women in developed countries, but meeting the DRI of zinc can be difficult, particularly if you don't eat meat. The use of supplements has at best a small effect on breast milk, but for the mother not eating zinc-rich foods, a zinc supplement may help maintain her zinc reserves. Recent studies suggest that an inadequate supply of zinc may be the cause of low vitamin A levels. Conversely, too much zinc can actually interfere with the absorption of copper.

Good sources of zinc: meat (beef, lamb, pork), poultry, seafood (oysters, crab, shrimp), eggs, seeds, legumes, yogurt, whole grains (zinc from whole grains may not be as well absorbed as that from other zinc sources), black-eyed peas, and wheat germ.

Iodine
You need only tiny amounts of this mineral, but without it your thyroid gland couldn't function. An iodine deficiency manifests itself as goiter, or enlarged thyroid gland. Iodine is part of the thyroid hormone that regulates body temperature and metabolism.

The DRI for iodine is set at 290 micrograms for breastfeeding women, and it requires almost no effort to meet this total. Iodine accumulates in direct proportion to the mother's diet. Breast milk generally contains about 178 micrograms in a liter, but one study found that iodine levels in human milk can be as high as 731 micrograms per liter. At that level, the nursing infant would be getting ten times his recommended intake. For this reason, mothers shouldn't take iodine supplements.

Good sources of iodine: iodized salt, seafood, plants, and animals that are fed plants.

Selenium
This trace mineral works with vitamin E to protect body compounds from damage. Selenium usually appears in breast milk at a concentration of 20 micrograms per liter. The DRI for breastfeeding mothers is 70 micrograms per day, up 10 micrograms from women not breastfeeding.

Increasing your intake of a nutrient usually does not boost the concentration of that nutrient in your breast milk. Selenium is an exception to this rule. The selenium content of food varies throughout the world. In Africa, mothers eating native foods, which are often low in selenium, had low selenium concentrations in their breast milk. A study of vegetarian mothers in California who eat local foods rich in selenium found that their breast milk had high concentrations of this mineral.

Mothers secrete about 12 to 20 micrograms of selenium in their breast milk each day, and their babies probably absorb 80 percent of that. As with many other nutrients, when you consume only about 1,800 calories a day, meeting the DRI of 70 micrograms of selenium can be tricky. Increase your intake to the 2,200-calorie range, and meeting your needs won't be so hard.

Good sources of selenium: seafood (including canned tuna), organ meats, and grains.

Biotin

Biotin is a B vitamin that has not yet been widely studied. We do know that it assists carbohydrates, proteins, and fats in getting their important jobs done. It is widely available in many foods, and biotin deficiency is extremely rare. The DRI for breastfeeding women is set at 35 micrograms.

There has been some concern that raw egg whites can bind and render useless the biotin you eat from other foods. While it is true that raw egg whites can bind with biotin, studies show that you'd have to eat about two dozen egg whites to get that effect. In any event, eating raw egg whites or whole uncooked eggs is not recommended because raw eggs may contain salmonella and cause serious illness in the person who eats them.

Good sources of biotin: egg yolk, yeast, liver, kidney, milk; some biotin is available in all plant and animal foods.

Pantothenic Acid

Pantothenic acid is a B vitamin that plays a small but vital role in energy metabolism. Though a deficiency in this nutrient is rare, it would manifest itself as vomiting, fatigue, insomnia, and perhaps diarrhea. The nutrient is abundant in so many foods that it's almost impossible not to get enough of it—any fatigue or insomnia you experience while breastfeeding is almost certainly not caused by a lack of pantothenic acid.

The DRI for pantothenic acid is 7 milligrams for nursing mothers. There have been no reports of deficiencies in breastfeeding mothers. Supplements can increase the content of pantothenic acid in breast milk. In one study, four mothers taking a pantothenic acid supplement of 1 milligram or more had significantly greater levels of pantothenic acid in their breast milk as compared to mothers who did not take supplements.

Good sources of pantothenic acid: meat, fish, poultry, whole grain cereals, and dried beans.

Copper

Copper helps make red blood cells, heals wounds, and forms part of the protective covering around nerves. Copper deficiency is quite rare. The DRI for copper is set at 1,300 micrograms per day to meet the needs of breastfeeding moms.

Animal studies show that copper is easily absorbed from breast milk, and so far there have been no case reports of any copper deficiency in breastfed babies. Furthermore, there does not appear to be a direct relationship between the amount of copper a mother eats and the level of copper in her breast milk. The copper concentration of breast milk naturally declines over the first four months of breastfeeding, at which time it levels off. Full-term healthy babies are born with a good supply of stored copper, and this reserve helps ensure that they have adequate copper available.

Good sources of copper: grains, nuts, organ meats, and seeds.

Manganese

This trace element works with your body's enzymes to help your metabolism function efficiently. The average adult woman has a reserve of only 18 milligrams in her entire body. The DRI for manganese is 2.6 milligrams daily. This nutrient is widely distributed in many foods.

Good sources of manganese: beans (chickpeas, black, soy), nuts, whole grain breads, cereals, wheat germ, and pineapple.

Fluoride

Fluoride builds stronger teeth and helps fight tooth decay. It also makes up part of your bones. Though it is present in the body in only small amounts, ensuring an adequate supply can almost guarantee healthier bones and teeth. Whenever the natural concentration of fluoride in local water supplies falls short of the desired level, supplements in the form of tablets or bottled fluoridated water are advised. In most cases your pediatrician can tell you if the local water supply contains fluoride.

Too much fluoride, which is a concern to some health advocates, can cause discoloring of the teeth. A day's supply of fluoridated water contains about 1 milligram of fluoride. The DRI for fluoride is 3 milligrams a day.

Breast milk contains about 16 micrograms of fluoride per liter. The fluoride level of mother's milk isn't easily increased by what a woman eats. In fact, when a large dose of fluoride (approximately three times the RDA) was given to one mother, it barely increased the fluoride concentration of her breast milk.

The question of when and how much to supplement fluoride for a breastfed baby concerns and puzzles doctors. In the April 25, 1990, issue of the *Journal of the American Medical Association,* Dr. John Greene of the University of California School of Dentistry addressed this issue in a response to a letter to the editor. Dr. Greene recommends that mothers and pediatricians follow the fluoridation guidelines set by the American Academy of Pediatrics (AAP), which state that infants should receive 0.25 milligrams of supplemental fluoride daily if their water supply contains less than 0.3 parts per million of fluoride. Currently the AAP Committee on Nutrition states it may not be necessary to give fluoride supplements to breastfed infants living in areas where the water is fluoridated. Check with your health care provider about fluoride recommendations.

Good sources of fluoride: drinking water (if naturally fluoridated), fluoride tablets, tea, and seafood.

Chromium

Chromium works with the hormone insulin to regulate your body's blood-sugar levels and to help release energy from glucose. The DRI is 44 to 45 micrograms daily. Chromium levels in breast milk are independent of the mother's food intake. Human breast milk contains approximately 50 micrograms of chromium per liter.

Good sources of chromium: whole grain bread and pasta, meat, poultry, fish, and most unrefined foods.

Molybdenum

Molybdenum sounds like something Superman might be afraid of. In fact, it's a trace element that makes up part of some essential enzymes in your body. We seem to need it in only minute amounts. Deficiencies of this nutrient are unknown, presumably because the amount we need is so small and isn't hard to obtain from food. The estimated DRI is 50 micrograms per day.

Good sources of molybdenum: seafood, meat, grains, nuts, and legumes.

4

PUTTING IT ALL TOGETHER—A MENU FOR MOTHERING

Having charts and lists of the nutrients you need is interesting, but it doesn't necessarily help you decide what to eat for breakfast. In this chapter you'll see what a good, healthy menu entails and find some simple dos and don'ts that will keep you and your baby happy.

Nursing mothers can eat three meals a day plus three or four healthy snacks. You need more food while you breastfeed, and you'll feel better if you eat frequently.

WHAT SHOULD I EAT?

While you are breastfeeding you want to make sure you get enough of all the important nutrients. Let your own natural hunger pangs be of some help. Eat when you're hungry, but try to eat good, healthy food. A vegetable salad with whole wheat bread on the side and some sliced chicken will provide you with many more nutrients than a Ring-Ding or Eskimo Pie.

There are certain foods you should try to eat every day (table 3).

Table 3. Outline of Your Daily Menu

A nursing mother needs to eat foods from all the six main food groups to meet her nutrient and calorie needs. The suggested daily servings are at the top, followed by a list of the foods in that group and the serving sizes of various foods.

Starch: **7–12 servings**

Bread, 1 slice	Baked beans, ¼ cup
Bagel, ¼	Beans (kidney, white, navy), ⅓ cup
Pasta, ⅓ cup	English muffin, ½
Cereal, ¾ cup	Rice, ⅓ cup

Protein: **7–8 ounces of beef, pork, lamb, veal, chicken, fish, turkey, or the equivalent. The foods below can be substituted for 1 ounce of meat.**

Egg, 1	Canned salmon, ¼ cup
Tofu, 4 ounces	Oysters, 6 medium
Cottage cheese, ¼ cup	Peanut butter, 1 tablespoon
Dried beans, ½ cup cooked	

Milk: **3–4 servings**

Milk, 1 cup	Yogurt, 8 ounces
Evaporated milk, ½ cup	Buttermilk, 1 cup
Tofu,* 1 cup	Soy milk,* 1 cup

Fruit: **3–6 servings. Choose at least one fruit rich in vitamin C (a citrus fruit is a good choice).**

Apple, 1	Peach, 1
Cherries, 12	Papaya, 1
Pineapple, ¾ cup	Orange juice, ½ cup
Orange, 1	

Vegetables: **3–5 servings. A serving is ½ cup of any cooked vegetable or vegetable juice or 1 cup of any raw vegetable. Choose a dark green leafy or vitamin A–rich veggie daily.**

Fat: 3–7 servings

Margarine or butter, 1 teaspoon	Diet margarine, 1 tablespoon
Mayonnaise, 1 teaspoon	Diet mayonnaise, 1 tablespoon
Cream, 1 tablespoon	Oil (olive and canola), 1 teaspoon

*Tofu is not traditionally placed in the milk group, but it can be a good calcium source for mothers who don't drink milk. Eight ounces (about 1 cup) of calcium-fortified tofu contains approximately 308 milligrams of calcium, 172 calories, 18 grams of vegetable protein, and 13 milligrams of iron. One cup of milk contains 300 milligrams of calcium, 90 to 160 calories, 8 grams of animal protein, and 0.12 milligrams of iron. Soy milk is also a good source of calcium.

If you eat the smaller number of recommended servings for all the food groups listed, select leaner meats, use 2 percent milk, and eat the portion sizes mentioned, the recommendations in table 3 add up to only 1,800 calories. A mother selecting the higher number of recommended servings will be eating about 2,700 calories. An intake of 1,800 calories is too low for most breastfeeding mothers—strive for a higher calorie intake.

HOW DO I KNOW IF MY DIET IS BALANCED?

To find out how well you are balancing your menu, write down everything you have to eat or drink for twenty-four hours. Include nighttime snacks and drinks. Review your twenty-four-hour menu and compare it to the food guide in table 3. Count foods only once; don't count cheese once in the milk group and once again in the meat group. Then answer these questions:

1. How many servings from the milk group did you have? ____
2. How many servings of meat, fish, chicken, cheese, or beans? _____

3. How many servings of fruit or fruit juices? _____

4. How many servings of vegetables? _____

5. How many servings of bread, cereal, rice, noodles, or other starches? _____

6. How many servings from the fat list? _____

7. How many "other" servings like soda, potato chips, cookies, jelly, and candy? _____

Add up your groups and compare to the recommended number of servings. If you are far under or over on any of the food groups, you may be lacking in some vital nutrients. Try to balance your menu by adjusting your food choices to meet the suggested number of servings in all six categories.

Mothers who need to increase their calorie intake can choose the higher calorie selections within a group. For example, if a mom chose to drink whole milk instead of skim milk, the calcium value would be almost the same but she'd eat 160 calories instead of the 80 in the nonfat milk. If she selected ⅓ cup of rice pilaf instead of an equal amount of plain rice, the calories would jump from 80 to 160.

Here are two different menus based on the six main food groups. They include all the recommended servings from every food group.

MENU ONE	MENU TWO
Breakfast	
Peanut butter on toast	Melted cheese on ½ English muffin
Sliced banana with yogurt	Small bowl of cereal with milk and fresh fruit
Coffee or tea	Coffee or tea
Snack	
Fruit and crackers	Fruited yogurt

Lunch

Chicken sandwich with
lettuce, tomato, and
mayonnaise
Milk

Vegetable and cheese pizza
Fruit cup

Snack

Mozzarella cheese stick
Sliced apple
Water or herb tea

Angel cake with yogurt

Water or herb tea

Supper

Baked fish
Roasted potato with
margarine
Steamed carrots
Salad with dressing
Milk

Vegetarian lasagna (made
with pasta, cheese,
spinach, and tomato)
Italian bread and margarine
Poached pears

Snack

Yogurt topped with cereal
and fresh fruit

Graham crackers and milk

The menus are quite different, but they both contain all the food groups mothers need. Portion sizes will determine the total calories and quantity of nutrients consumed. Mothers who want a more detailed guide to portions should refer to chapter 6.

CULTURAL DIFFERENCES

Not all mothers eat the same foods. Women of Asian or Hispanic heritage might select foods that are quite different from those on the menu of a woman of European background. Even though the foods are different, they can still be combined to provide a balanced, healthy menu. However, Hispanic or Asian-American mothers eating traditional diets may need to pay special attention to certain nutrients. Asian diets generally contain few dairy foods. A nursing mother eating a traditional Chinese or Asian diet will want to select foods such as tofu, bok choy, mustard greens, and calcium-fortified fruit juices to meet her calcium needs. One nutrition study found that Chinese American adults did not consume enough folic acid, zinc, calcium, vitamins A and C, and iron to meet the recommended levels for these nutrients. Nursing mothers who eat traditional Chinese American menus will want to make sure they get foods that contain these nutrients.

Young Mexican-American mothers eating traditional Mexican foods while breastfeeding have been found to have diets that are low in iron, vitamin A, and calcium. To boost calcium, mothers should be encouraged to eat low-fat cheeses and milk. Café con leche, a drink that is equal parts milk and coffee, can boost calcium, as can chocolate milk and hot chocolate. (Mothers don't want to drink more than two full cups of coffee a day because of its potential stimulating effect on their babies and because it might interfere with the mother's iron absorption.) Eating lean red meats will help boost iron. Red chilis in Mexican-style foods can be an excellent source of vitamin A.

MOTHERS SHOULD EAT THREE MEALS PLUS SNACKS

Eating frequently can actually help control hunger and overeating. Snacks that contain protein, complex carbohydrate, and some fat help keep your blood-sugar levels steady. Eating enough food allows fat cells to make the hormone leptin, and leptin signals the hypothalamus to cut our appetite and make us feel full. When the stomach is empty it makes another hormone called ghrelin. Ghrelin signals to the brain that the body needs more food and we become hungry again. If you skip meals or snacks, you may confuse this internal appetite-regulating system. You'll also feel weak, famished, and tired. It may sound crazy but hunger is the enemy of anyone who wants to eat well and lose weight. It leads to overeating and poor food choices. Just observe the quality of what you eat when you are "starving." That is when mothers overconsume because they are too hungry to make good choices.

Snacks that are rich in simple sugars like candy, sweetened fruit juice, and soda are rapidly digested. These foods give a boost to your blood sugar. Your body may be overproducing insulin, the hormone responsible for keeping your blood sugar steady. When too much insulin is produced, it can bring your blood sugar low enough to cause a new round of hunger. To prevent this cycle, simply eat regularly and eat foods like whole grains, fruit, vegetables, lean meats, and low-fat cheeses for snacks. Snacking on fruit, vegetables, cheese sticks, and yogurt tends to be filling and self-limiting, whereas "dry" salty foods like chips, pretzels, and crackers never quite lead to fullness because they contain very little water. Foods that have high water content tend to promote fullness.

One word of warning about nighttime snacking. If you need to eat something at the 2:00 A.M. feeding because you're really hungry, then by all means have something to eat. But keep in mind that nighttime snacking can be a tough habit to break once you're no longer nursing and don't need the extra food.

DO I HAVE TO EAT BREAKFAST?

I think all breastfeeding mothers should eat in the morning. If you have gone all night without food, your body needs some refueling. Breakfast doesn't have to be bacon and eggs with a side order of hash browns. It can be much easier—and lower in fat.

Cereal is my favorite breakfast food because it's quick and nutritious. The added milk provides protein and calcium and the cereal itself is a rich source of B vitamins and zinc. Top it with fruit or drink a glass of juice and you've started yourself off on the right foot. (Unless you're eating a very large bowl of cereal—and some of us do—you'll probably need a side order of toast with it, too.)

A good breakfast gives you about 25 percent of the energy and nutrition you need for the day, but I think it does even more. The habit of eating breakfast will serve you well long after you stop breastfeeding. People who lose weight and successfully keep it off report eating breakfast. Many people have more energy in the morning if they eat breakfast, and as we get older, breakfast seems to help in the fight against overeating and weight gain.

WHY DOES EATING BREAKFAST MAKE ME EVEN HUNGRIER?

I often hear this question from adults who are trying to control their weight. The answer may be that you are eating the wrong foods. When Dr. David Ludwig served overweight teenagers three different breakfasts, he found that the kids ate less when they had a protein-rich breakfast compared to a breakfast of processed cereal. He served each teen an egg-white omelet rich in protein on one day. The next breakfast was an old-fashioned oatmeal made with whole, not processed, "steel cut" oats. At the third meal he served them a more refined packaged oatmeal. After each breakfast he assessed how much they ate later in the day. The kids ate most when they were served a breakfast of packaged oatmeal. If you feel hungry after your usual breakfast, reexamine what you are eating. Avoid foods with a lot of sugar and try something with protein in it such as an egg, milk, or yogurt, and include a fruit or vegetable. And remember, hunger is normal while breastfeeding. You're the sole source of nourishment for your baby and you must eat enough for him, too. Listen to the signals your body is sending and do the best you can to make food choices that carry the most nutrition.

HOW MUCH WATER DO I NEED?

While you're breastfeeding you need to drink more fluids—at least two quarts every day. It doesn't have to be only water. Fruit juice, tea, and milk can all help to satisfy your need for fluids. Even fruits and vegetables contain significant amounts of water.

A mother produces about 23 ounces of milk for her baby every day. You must replace those 23 ounces and take in extra fluid to meet your own body's needs. Water prevents dehydration, but it also helps to eliminate the body wastes created during metabolism. Water dilutes these wastes so that they can be excreted from your body more easily.

It's frequently suggested that lots of extra water is needed to make breast milk and that if a mother needs to increase the volume of her milk she should drink more fluids. This is not true. Drinking more water does not make a mother produce more milk. Recently, nineteen healthy mothers and their babies participated in a study to measure the impact fluids have on breast-milk production. The nursing mothers in the study increased their fluid intake by over 30 percent, but there was no resulting increase in milk production. Forced drinking may be detrimental to milk production, even diminishing the amount produced.

Mothers who drink lots of water will urinate more often and have lighter-color urine. Mothers who don't drink the recommended amounts will still produce an adequate supply of milk, but they will urinate less often and probably complain of constant thirst.

Most mothers can rely on their thirst to tell them when they need more fluids. Drink as soon as you feel the first thirst sensations. One good way to get enough fluids is to take a drink of water every time you nurse your baby. Remember that when it is very hot, your need for liquids increases; make sure you drink a bit more in hot weather.

My sister Sheila gave me a great tip. Before you go to bed, fill a tall glass with ice cubes. Place it in the baby's room or wherever you nurse during the night. When the baby wakes for her nighttime feeding, the ice will have melted and you'll have a cold, refreshing glass of water to drink while the baby nurses.

WHAT FOODS SHOULD I AVOID?

Many mothers think they must survive on a bland diet while nursing. This isn't true. Mothers from many cultures breastfeed successfully on diets that are far different from ours. Feel free to use any seasonings you like. Using salt does not increase the sodium in your breast milk, and pepper won't make your milk spicy. Some foods do bother mothers; you can read more about this in chapter 8. The substances you do need to be careful with are alcohol and coffee. In general, limit coffee to two cups a day and alcohol to an occasional drink (more about this in chapter 8, too).

WHAT IS MOST IMPORTANT?

Don't focus on what you shouldn't eat. Instead emphasize all the good foods you *can* have. Calcium, zinc, magnesium, vitamin B_6, and folic acid are the nutrients you need the most. To get them, you'll want to eat whole grain cereals and grains, lots of green leafy vegetables, poultry, seafood, milk, cheese, yogurt, and lean cuts of meat. Not a bad way to lose weight, when you come to think of it!

5

THE NATURE OF
MOTHERS' DIETS

At some point while you're nursing, you may be interested in losing weight. Losing weight while you're breastfeeding is a completely different proposition than it was before you had your baby. This chapter will explain what to expect from your body as you lose weight and what is safe and what isn't.

HOW I GOT INTERESTED IN THIS SUBJECT

When I was pursuing my education in nutrition I was fortunate enough to have been accepted into an intensive thirteen-month training program at the Boston Lying-in Hospital, now known as the Brigham and Women's Hospital. The Boston Lying-in was a Harvard Medical School hospital that at the time delivered more babies than any other hospital in Boston. It was here that I first got to talk to new moms about their diets.

Our hospital was filled with women: some were in for surgery or tests, but most were new mothers. One of my regular assignments was to speak to every new breastfeeding mother about the role that good nutrition plays in a satisfying nursing experience. Of course, eight out of ten new mothers wanted to know how they could safely lose weight and still breastfeed their babies. No problem, I told them—one of the big extra bonuses of breastfeeding is that you can lose weight even while eating 2,700 calories a day.

In 1978, it was thought that nursing women could lose weight effortlessly because they needed so many calories to make milk and keep the baby well fed. This notion of automatic weight loss certainly seemed to make sense, and it was backed by the National Academy of Sciences.

Years later, a new study suggested that all mothers would probably not automatically lose weight if they ate the 2,700 calories being recommended for breastfeeding mothers. This study, published by Dr. Nancy Butte, found that breastfeeding mothers could successfully nurse their babies on far fewer calories than were usually recommended. I couldn't help but think that there were mothers all over Boston who were having trouble losing weight and would love to get their hands on that friendly dietitian trainee who told them to eat as much as they wanted.

CAN'T I JUST ENJOY BEING A MOM FOR A WHILE?

When I started writing this chapter, I had a conversation with my good friend Marta about weight loss. Marta has a four-year-old daughter, and our families have been friends since we met in a postpartum exercise class four years ago. "I think it's awful that mothers are pressured into losing weight while they breastfeed. It's as if we're no good unless we're skinny. For goodness sake, we just had a baby and then we start to criticize ourselves for being overweight. Nobody bugs the fathers if they've put on a few pounds."

Marta's comments reflect the way a lot of mothers feel. There is tremendous pressure to be the "perfect" woman. Ads in magazines show skinny models who are on the edge of malnutrition. Ads on TV show skinny mothers who hold their tiny babies while they promote liquid diets. The not-so-subtle message is to strive for the media idea of perfection.

This book is not about being skinny and malnourished. It's about eating good food—enough to take care of you and your child—and obtaining a weight through proper food that is best for your long-term health. Don't do anything you don't feel good about. The last thing I want to do is add more pressure to a new mother's busy life. Raising and nursing a child is the most important job you can do.

If a breastfeeding mother wants to nurse and lose weight, too, then the information in these chapters will help her meet her goals safely. If she doesn't want to lose weight, she can use the information to make sure she eats the foods that are essential to the good health of her and her child.

WOMEN, OBESITY, AND HEALTH

Approximately 50 percent of American women are defined as being overweight or obese. Overweight is defined as having a body mass index (BMI) above 25 (see page 222 to plot your BMI). Addressing weight right after pregnancy is a good idea for two reasons. The first is that most of us have weight to lose and the second is now, as we create a new family lifestyle, we should be laying the foundation for positive food habits. It's much easier to prevent a weight problem than to treat it later on. Researchers in Wisconsin have found that women who lost most of their pregnancy weight by their babies' six-month birthdays gained about five pounds over the next eight years, but women who did not return to their prepregnancy weight gained about eighteen pounds over the same number of years. Interestingly, of the 795 women in this study, those who breastfed their baby and exercised regularly had significantly lower weight gains with time, suggesting that the combination of exercise and breastfeeding may be beneficial in long-term weight control.

The Nurses Health Study is an ongoing research project of the

Division of Preventive Medicine at Brigham and Women's Hospital in Boston. This prospective cohort study followed the weight and health risks of 115,000 female nurses over a sixteen-year period. The nurses who gained more than twenty-two pounds since age eighteen were at greater risk of developing heart disease. Obesity is also linked to other health problems like diabetes, high blood pressure, high cholesterol, asthma, arthritis, and overall poor health. Weight loss is not just about good looks. Your good health is at issue, too. A diet that keeps you in the range of your desirable weight is also more likely to have a lower percentage of fat and contain lots of good, nutritious foods.

WHY LOSING WEIGHT WHILE BREASTFEEDING IS SO DIFFERENT

Giving birth and breastfeeding bring physical and emotional changes. Breastfeeding affects what you need to eat, and being a new mother reduces the time you have for cooking. Most new mothers complain of constant fatigue and an inability to accomplish anything: "I was home all day with the baby. I never put my feet up once, but I don't feel like I got anything done." You simply don't have the time or energy to follow complex dieting plans. In a study conducted at the University of California, Dr. Mary Wilson Blackburn asked twelve women to keep food and activity diaries while pregnant and while breastfeeding. The diaries revealed that once the mothers delivered their babies and were nursing, they spent 10 to 15 percent less time resting than they did while pregnant. The time lost to Mom was spent on taking care of the new baby. So again, if you feel tired and don't have time to take care of yourself, you're not alone.

The good news is that proper nutrition can help prevent fatigue. Before becoming a mother, a woman might have been able to lose weight by skipping meals or just drinking liquids to cut calories. These strategies won't work now. If you curb your food intake too severely you won't get enough nutrition to maintain your proper energy level. A mother on a severely restricted diet can develop problems with her milk supply, especially in the first few weeks after delivery as you begin to produce milk. In general the mother's diet is not related to milk volume, and if you think you are not making enough milk it is probably due to poor suckling or not enough time at the breast rather than inadequate milk supply. But not eating enough will definitely make you tired and add to the fatigue that comes automatically with having the demands of a new baby. To prevent exhaustion, you must eat enough to keep your energy reserves fueled. Eating on a regular, predictable schedule not only ensures adequate energy, it is also the most successful way to manage your weight. People (including new mothers) who stick to a schedule feel better and lose weight faster than those who skip meals.

Your need for nutrition is greater now than at any other time in your life. Perhaps you lost weight before by eliminating breads, starches, or even dairy products. If you do that now, you may be restricting your intake of nutrients such as calcium and the B vitamins like thiamine. In most cases, if you don't eat enough of the essential nutrients, your body will automatically steal them from its own reserves, directing them to your breast milk so that your baby will be well nourished. This diversion of vitamins and minerals is fine if it happens only occasionally, but a continuous depletion of your own body stores could cause you health problems later on. Some researchers even believe that a mother's reserves may not always be adequate to compensate for her inadequate intake of nutrients.

The good news about breastfeeding is that you probably can eat more than you are normally accustomed to and still lose weight. Studies suggest that all new mothers won't be able to lose weight eating the full 2,700 calories recommended in government tables, but most women eating 2,200 calories a day can lose weight. Those 2,200 calories are a lot more satisfying than the 1,200 calories most women restrict themselves to when dieting.

GO SLOW

While you breastfeed, you should lose weight more slowly than you would otherwise. Safe weight loss for most adult women when not nursing is thought to be one to two pounds per week, or about eight pounds a month. For breastfeeding moms, safe weight loss after the first postpartum month is thought to be only one to two pounds a month for the first four to six months, and not more than four and a half pounds a month after that.

For many of you, one to two pounds a month may sound painfully slow. But remember, you won't be depriving yourself, so you shouldn't feel hungry. If you nurse your baby for ten months, it could add up to a loss of ten to twenty pounds!

HOW THE WEIGHT COMES OFF

Weight loss is greatest between three and six months postpartum. The average weight loss is one to two pounds per month, though overweight women may lose four to five pounds in a month. After the first month, rapid weight loss greater than four to five pounds is not advised. In an Australian study of 174 mothers, weight loss was found to level off by the sixth month.

Many women are unable to reach their prepregnancy weight until they stop nursing altogether. As long as you breastfeed, your breasts will add at least one to three pounds to the scale.

EXERCISE—IT'S DIFFERENT, TOO

How much exercise and energy you use in a day changes considerably when you become a mother. Taking care of and feeding a child usually involves more housework and family chores, but this is rarely the kind of activity that burns calories. Many mothers find that being housebound with a new baby considerably curtails their activity levels. A small study of American women showed that sedentary breastfeeding moms used up only 1,800 to 1,900 calories in a day's activities (this did not include the calories they used to make breast milk). A comparison group of non-breastfeeding mothers performing light to moderate activities burned up 2,200 calories.

This does not mean that all breastfeeding mothers burn fewer calories. If you are chasing around other busy toddlers or working in a strenuous job or even putting in a summer garden, your energy expenditure can be far greater than the 1,800 calories mentioned. In fact, in one study mothers exercising on a regular basis were able to expend 2,600 calories daily, and that did not include the approximately 500 calories used to make breast milk. Read more about the benefits of exercise in chapter 7.

The bottom line is that while nursing you must be prudent about how you diet. There just isn't as much leeway in your nutritional needs. I'm a firm believer in taking it slowly. Lose weight by selecting food carefully; let the extra calories needed to breast-feed come from your own fat reserves. That way you burn fat while you eat nutritious foods and keep healthy.

POSTPREGNANCY WEIGHT LOSS

You're not alone if you expected to return to your prepregnancy weight once you delivered. Keep in mind that it took your body nine months to build your baby's first home. For many moms, it takes as long or longer to return to their prepregnancy size.

It can be helpful to understand where you kept the extra weight you carried while you were pregnant. If you had the textbook pregnancy and weren't overweight before you got pregnant, then you should have gained twenty-five to thirty-five pounds. If you were underweight before conception, your doctor may have encouraged you to gain twenty-eight to forty pounds or more. An overweight mom could have had a perfectly healthy baby and pregnancy with a weight gain of fifteen to twenty-five pounds. Table 4 shows how those theoretical pounds would have been distributed.

Table 4. How Did I Gain So Much and Where Did It Go?

Infant	7.5–8.5 pounds
Placenta and umbilical cord	1.5 pounds
Increase in mother's blood volume	4 pounds
Increase in mother's uterus	2 pounds
Increase in breast tissue	1 pound
Amniotic fluid that surrounds baby	1.8 pounds
Mother's fat/protein stores	7.5 pounds
Tissue fluids	2.7 pounds
Total	28–29 pounds

Once your baby was born, there was an immediate drop in weight caused by the delivery of the baby and the expulsion of the placenta. Since the baby was no longer relying on your blood supply, your own blood volume and fluid levels began to return to normal. You may have noticed you had to urinate more frequently while your body got rid of some unneeded fluid. Some women may temporarily retain fluid longer, and they may find that if they step on the scale they won't have lost as much weight as they expected.

There are no hard-and-fast rules about weight loss after birth, but one hour after delivery the average mother can expect to lose about thirteen and a half pounds. Between the first hour and twelfth day postpartum, another three and a half pounds should disappear. By the sixth week, any weight left above the prepregnancy level is fat and breast tissue.

HOW MUCH WEIGHT IS IT SAFE TO LOSE—AND HOW FAST?

Most breastfeeding mothers lose about one to two pounds per month over the first six months. This seems to be a normal and safe amount. A weight loss exceeding four and a half pounds per month is not recommended. Women who gain more during their pregnancy lose more postpartum and probably need to. When Cheryl Lovelady, Ph.D., R.D., a nutrition researcher, wanted to determine if weight loss while breastfeeding was safe for the baby, she asked forty overweight nursing moms to help answer the question. The mothers were asked to be in one of two groups. One group restricted calories by approximately 500 and exercised four times per week. The other group was asked to maintain their usual diet and limit exercise to once a week. The diet and exercise moms lost about one pound per week and the researchers concluded that exclusively breastfeeding moms losing about one pound per week did not affect the growth of their infants.

But postpregnancy weight loss is highly unpredictable, with wide fluctuations from one mother to another. I was surprised when five days after the delivery of my eight-pound, twelve-ounce baby girl the scale showed I had lost only eleven pounds. Don't be too disappointed when your body doesn't instantly return to its prepregnancy shape. Don't be discouraged either if you must still wear maternity clothes to feel comfortable. Just take care of yourself—don't push weight loss now. In fact, don't even get serious about losing weight until at least six weeks after delivery.

WHAT IF I LOSE WEIGHT TOO FAST?

If you are losing weight too fast (more than four and a half pounds per month after the first month), then you really aren't eating all you should. Your total food intake isn't adequate, and therefore your intake of nutrients probably isn't adequate, either. Milk production will probably not be affected, but you will be tired and irritable and the nursing and parenting experience might be more stressful.

WHAT DO I NEED TO BE CAREFUL ABOUT?

The risk associated with an overzealous and too restrictive weight loss plan is that you may compromise your milk supply. In a study of short-term calorie restriction of breastfeeding mothers, Margaret Strode and coworkers at the Department of Pediatrics, University of California, Davis, discovered that when a small group of nursing mothers restricted their daily intake of calories from an average of 2,300 to about 1,600, there was no immediate change in their babies' weight gain or feeding schedule. In the week that followed the calorie restriction, however, there was a measurable difference. The babies did not take in as much milk, they fed less often, and their rate of weight gain decreased. While mothers who strictly limit their calorie intake might see no immediate effect on their milk production, there may be repercussions in the days that follow.

Short-term fasting does not seem to harm milk production. Two studies of mothers fasting from fourteen and a half to twenty hours found that there was no difference in milk secretion. This might be important for mothers who must fast for a short while for a medical test or for religious reasons.

CAN I USE LIQUID DRINKS OR DIET PILLS WHILE NURSING?

Liquid diets and weight loss medications are not recommended for nursing mothers. Some over-the-counter appetite suppressants control hunger with massive amounts of caffeine. If you use these products you can transfer the caffeine to your baby, possibly making him irritable and fussy. Do not use "natural" weight loss supplements. None of them are proven to be effective and some, like ephedra, have been banned by the FDA because they are dangerous.

In the May 1991 issue of *American Baby* magazine, Gail Kaitschuck, L.D., R.D., tells the story of a new mother who used an over-the-counter high-protein drink to lose the extra forty pounds she gained while pregnant. She started the liquid diet two weeks postpartum, while nursing her baby. Three weeks later she and the baby were hospitalized: the baby for failure to thrive because of inadequate milk supply and the mother for fatigue and low blood pressure. Both baby and mother were harmed because the liquid protein drink didn't meet the energy requirements for a breastfeeding mother. Liquid protein diets are simply inappropriate as an exclusive feeding for any breastfeeding mother. A liquid meal replacement can be a quick and useful item to keep on hand when you have no time to cook. Just make sure it has a good source of protein and include real food, too. Read about "Meals in a Blender" in chapter 10.

WHEN SHOULD I START A DIET?

The Subcommittee on Nutrition During Lactation suggests that mothers not start weight loss diets until at least two to three weeks after they give birth, since curtailing calories any earlier might be detrimental to the nursing experience. The first few weeks of breastfeeding are important for establishing an adequate milk supply and for ensuring a good bond between you and your baby. I think new mothers should take at least six weeks before taking on any new challenges, including dieting.

IS IT NORMAL TO LOSE WEIGHT WHILE BREASTFEEDING?

Yes, most mothers lose one or two pounds per month while breastfeeding. A mother who is overweight should be able to lose up to one and a quarter pounds a week without adversely affecting her milk production. But not all nursing women will automatically lose weight.

When I reviewed the research about weight loss and breastfeeding, I found several cases in which weight loss was quite slow or even nonexistent. In 1989, Dr. Marie Brewer reported the results of a study of the weight loss patterns of fifty-six new mothers. Twenty-one were exclusively breastfeeding, fifteen were exclusively formula feeding, and twenty were breastfeeding and using formula. The women's weights and measurements were taken within the first two days after they gave birth, then again at three and six months postpartum. There was no significant difference in the rate of weight loss between any of the groups of mothers. Those with lower pregnancy weights were likely to have greater weight loss. The mothers feeding formula to their babies ate a lot fewer calories than the breastfeeding mothers, but very few of the nursing mothers ate the recommended 2,700 calories a day, either. Breastfeeding is touted as a way to lose weight effortlessly but when compared to weight loss of new mothers feeding their babies formula, the breastfeeding moms do not automatically have an easier time losing weight. A Canadian study that compared the weight loss of 236 breastfeeding and formula-feeding mothers found that at nine months after delivery the type of feeding did not significantly predict how much the mothers would lose. But in another study, this time in 110 women followed from 2 weeks to 18 months postpartum, the breastfeeding mothers were found to have more weight loss, although the researchers were quick to state that the difference was minimal. At the University of California researchers found that weight loss could be traced to breastfeeding when women nursed for at least six months, and when the hip measurements of twenty-four women at six months postpartum were measured in a Massachusetts study, the breastfeeding moms had greater weight loss around their hips than the women who were not breastfeeding.

Carolyn Manning-Dalton at the University of Connecticut weighed twenty-seven women twelve days after giving birth. They weighed, on average, thirteen pounds above their prepregnancy weight. Over a subsequent three months, these mothers averaged a weight loss of approximately four and a half pounds while eating about 2,200 calories a day. The authors of this study concluded that breastfeeding does not automatically promote weight loss, and they suggest that the recommended 2,700 calories a day is more than most nursing mothers need.

The Stockholm Pregnancy and Weight Development Study is a prospective study of body weight changes in 1,423 women. The study is designed to identify predictors of postpartum weight retention. Women in the study who were most likely to return to their prepregnancy weight were found to eat a regular lunch and supper most often. The women with the greatest weight retention at one year postpartum were found to eat more calories during their pregnancy as well as after, they increased their snacking after pregnancy to three times per day, and they decreased their frequency of regular lunch meals. Women who retained more than ten pounds were less active compared to the smaller women. The strongest predictor for weight retention was how much mothers gained while pregnant; women who gained more than the recommended amount had a harder time getting it off. Older mothers also retained more weight than younger moms. There were large variations in weight gains and losses, but the bottom line was that breastfeeding alone does not guarantee weight loss and that lifestyle habits including activity and regular meals had a significant impact on weight.

It has also been reported that women can actually gain weight while nursing. In the Stockholm study 30 percent of the women lost weight, 56 percent stayed about the same or gained a little, and 14 percent gained ten pounds. Of course, if a mother is below ideal body weight, weight gain is fine, but it could be a problem if she is overweight.

What can you expect? You'll probably lose some weight while you breastfeed, but you may not automatically shed all of the weight you put on while you were pregnant. Good food choices and a plan to eat well can help you lose those last pounds steadily without compromising your health or your nursing experience.

HOW MANY CALORIES DO NEW MOMS REALLY NEED?

For years the answer has been: a healthy mother who gained the recommended amount of weight while pregnant needs an additional 500 calories per day while she nurses her baby, and underweight mothers might need 650 additional calories. Add these numbers to the 2,200 calories believed necessary for all women age fifteen to fifty and the total is 2,700 to 2,850 calories a day while you are breastfeeding. The figure of 500 extra calories per day for all nursing mothers was calculated by the Food and Nutrition Board, a division of the National Academy of Sciences Institute of Medicine. It is estimated that the average mother makes about 750 milliliters of breast milk every day. It takes an additional 640 calories to make this milk. Approximately 100 to 150 of these calories are expected to come from the fat that you stored while you were pregnant. That leaves 500 calories you need to supply from food. Women who did not eat enough extra food to meet the requirement of 2,700 to 2,850 calories per day were thought to be at risk of jeopardizing their own health and possibly compromising their ability to breastfeed their babies.

Though these calculations look good on paper, they may not hold true for all of us when we actually try to plan out calorie levels that allow for good nutrition and reasonable weight loss. In fact, recent research suggests that if some of us were to follow these recommendations, we might still be carrying around our pregnancy fat at our baby's first birthday.

In 1984, Dr. Nancy Butte, an expert on nutrition and lactation at the Children's Nutrition Research Center at Baylor College of Medicine in Texas, published a study that changed the way we think about calories during breastfeeding. She found that mothers were able to nurse their babies successfully and lose weight while consuming fewer than the 2,700 calories a day specified in the RDA.

Dr. Butte studied the diets of forty-five breastfeeding mothers over a period of four months. These women were able to successfully nurse their babies while eating an average of only 2,186 calories. They were also able to lose an average of eleven pounds in the four months of the study. The 2,186 calories is more than 500 calories below the RDA for breastfeeding mothers.

There are three possible reasons Dr. Butte's study came up with a different calorie level than the RDA. First, not all women produce the theoretical 750 milliliters of milk a day. In this study, the women produced only 735 milliliters, or 25 ounces, of milk. Second, breast milk is thought to contain 67 to 77 calories per 100 milliliters. In Dr. Butte's study, it averaged only 64 calories per 100 milliliters. Finally, the base level of 2,200 calories needed each day by nonpregnant women may be too high to begin with.

Breastfeeding women probably need an extra 330 to 450 calories daily above the number needed when not breastfeeding. This is about the same amount of food needed as in the second and third trimester of pregnancy. Overweight women may not need the full 330 to 450 calories, but no nursing mother should go below a total calorie intake of 1,800.

Another factor influencing caloric needs is that nursing mothers may use calories more efficiently. Dr. P. J. Illingworth studied nineteen healthy new mothers. Twelve were breastfeeding and seven were bottle-feeding. Seven nonpregnant, nonlactating women participated as controls. The study, published in a 1985 issue of the *British Medical Journal*, examined how breastfeeding mothers utilize calories. He found that breastfeeding enhances a woman's metabolic efficiency and that new mothers may not need to increase their calorie intake to the level that is currently recommended. This means that some women may be more energy-sparing and that individual hormones and activity play a part in energy needs.

As you can see, deciding how many calories you need while breastfeeding isn't simple. The current recommendation for mothers who want to breastfeed is still about 2,700 calories per day; at the very least, mothers are advised to eat 1,800 calories a day. This recommendation was suggested by the Subcommittee on Nutrition During Lactation and published in *Nutrition During Lactation* in 1991, and it still stands today. The 2,700-calorie level probably guarantees an adequate diet, assuming the mother makes reasonable food choices. But as the research studies suggest, 2,700 calories may be too much for some mothers and may cause weight gain or prevent weight loss. The ideal approach is to tailor to your individual needs. This can be done by eating three meals, including all the important food groups, and losing weight at an acceptable level. The next chapter will introduce you to a more individual approach.

Don't automatically assume you should cut down to the 1,800-calorie level. Mothers eating only 1,800 calories a day must pay very close attention to getting adequate supplies of calcium, zinc, magnesium, vitamin B_6, and folic acid. It is important for mothers to realize that when calories are restricted, food is restricted and nutrients may be harder to get. This is the time you need to be well nourished, so plan menus carefully. Because the research and data on what breastfeeding mothers really need to eat aren't entirely clear, don't rely completely on what the doctors or scientists recommend. Instead, listen to your own body and come up with a personal plan for healthy eating. Lifestyle and food habits will be essential to weight control all your life. Eat enough so that you feel good and your baby is happy, but don't feel compelled to stuff yourself. Again, the next chapter will help you make the healthful food choices that will be best for you and your baby.

6

A NATURAL DIET FOR MOTHERS

Your goal while breastfeeding is to eat enough food to keep you healthy and satisfied. On the pages that follow I'll give you enough information to let you eat well, lose weight gently, and have a happy nursing experience.

The dietary system I use incorporates nine food groups. Use the food groups and suggested menus that follow to make decisions about what to eat and to guide you in planning healthy meals. You should eat well but allow your body to do what it is supposed to do: use up the fat you stored while pregnant. Just as breastfeeding is the natural continuation of pregnancy, gentle weight loss can be the natural course of events while breastfeeding.

WILL I BE ON A DIET?

I don't like to use the word *diet* because it sounds as if you'll have to change your eating habits just long enough to reach the dress size you envision. Once you reach that weight goal, you'll feel you can indulge in all the "forbidden" foods again. That's not the way to ensure healthy, permanent weight loss. Please don't think of this as a "diet" if that means short-term change. Instead, think of it as a time to take stock of your eating habits and make some permanent changes for the better.

You now have a family and the meal style and habits you create today will lay the foundation for the future. All you need to do is take care of yourself; eat three meals, include proper snacks, and the weight and energy will take care of themselves. The following pages will suggest what to include at those meals and snack times.

HOW MUCH CAN I EAT?

My Natural Diet for Mothers is like no other diet you've been on. Instead of being based on deprivation, this menu is meant to meet your calorie needs and satisfy your appetite. In fact, you may feel like you have never eaten so much food before. You're probably right.

Remember that, on average, mothers secrete 420 to 700 calories each day in their breast milk and that it takes even more calories to make that milk. Without even increasing your activity, your body will need many more calories than you are probably accustomed to. Also the foods that I encourage are packed with nutrition but are low in fat and empty calories. I might recommend that you eat the equivalent of three slices of bread, three ounces of protein, a serving of fruit and vegetables, and a cup of yogurt for lunch. These foods are rich in the B vitamins, calcium, and folic acid that mothers need, but they add up to only 500 calories. A quarter-pound hamburger with cheese, French fries, and Coke would give you close to 1,000 calories without being as rich in some important nutrients.

As far as I'm concerned, there isn't a single food you can't have, no matter how rich in calories, fat, or sugar. (The only exception would be foods or drinks high in alcohol or caffeine.) It's not the one candy bar or the occasional piece of birthday cake that gets you into trouble. It's your whole pattern of eating that counts.

WHERE DO I START?

Begin by reading the one-day sample menu. The food is distributed in three meals and three snacks. If you eat at the high end of the portions you'll be taking in about 2,700 calories. A more individualized plan can be developed, as I'll show you later in this chapter.

HOW DO I USE THE NATURAL DIET FOR MOTHERS?

Follow the meal plan and menu guide in this chapter to make smart eating choices. If you need to modify the caloric content, just follow the adaptation guidelines I give in the discussions of the individual food groups.

A NATURAL DIET FOR MOTHERS

At no other time in your life will you be likely to eat so much and still expect to lose weight. To balance your caloric needs with your nutrient needs, eat the following number of servings daily from the six main food groups:

Nonfat milk	3–4
Protein	2 servings (7–9 ounces)
Vegetables	4–5
Fruit	4–6
Starch	7–12
Fat	5–7

These six categories are the key to a healthy diet. My system adds three other groups as well: free group, combination group, and the daily option group of foods to eat only once a day. The free, combination, and daily option foods add flavor and variety to your meals, but they aren't nutrition powerhouses.

In order for a food to be placed in a category, it must be similar in the amount of calories, carbohydrate, protein, fat, vitamins, and minerals to the other foods in the group. Portions are designed so that every food in a group will have the same number of calories per serving. For example, one slice of bread has approximately 80 calories, as does one half of an English muffin. These two foods from the starch group can be substituted for each other without increasing or decreasing the calories in a meal.

The food groups can appear a bit confusing at first, but read through them, work with them a bit, and you'll find they are extremely useful. Using these nine food groups, a mother might come up with the following menu for a day's meals. This menu gives her the recommended amounts of calories and nutrients, provides plenty to eat, and tastes good, too.

One Day's Sample Menu

Food Group	Amount	Sample Food
		Breakfast
Milk	1	1 cup nonfat milk
Protein	1	1 egg, poached
Fruit	1–2	½–1 cup orange juice
Starch	1–3	1–3 slices toast
Fat	1–2	1–2 teaspoons margarine
Free	—	Coffee/tea

10:00 A.M.
Snack

Food Group	Amount	Sample Food
Milk	½	½ cup yogurt
Starch	1	¾ cup corn flakes
Fruit	1	½ banana, sliced

Lunch

Milk	1	1 cup milk
Protein	3	3 ounces sliced chicken
Starch	2	1 roll
Vegetable	2	1 tomato, sliced, and 1 cup salad
Fat	1–3	1–2 teaspoons mayonnaise and 1 tablespoon salad dressing

2:00 P.M. Snack

Protein	1	1 tablespoon peanut butter
Starch	1	3 graham crackers
Fruit	1–2	½–1 cup grapefruit juice
Vegetable	1	½ cup vegetable sticks

Supper

Milk	1	1 cup nonfat milk
Protein	3	3 ounces cooked steak
Vegetable	2	½ cup carrots, ½ cup green beans
Starch	1–3	½–1½ cups cooked noodles
Fat	1–2	1–2 teaspoons margarine
Fruit	1	1 peach

9:00 P.M. Snack

Milk	½	½ cup milk
Starch	1	¾ cup cereal

Because foods in the lists are grouped by their caloric and nutritional profiles, you might be surprised where some of them turn up. For instance, cheese is in the meat group because it contains protein and has similar calorie content as meat foods. Corn and potatoes are very rich in carbohydrate, so they find their niche in the starch group, not the vegetable group. A food like pizza will be found in the combination food group since it is made up of starch (crust), protein (cheese), and fat (oil). If vegetables top that pizza, then a serving from the vegetable group would be added, too.

My meal plans use nonfat milk. Nonfat milk has the same calcium value as whole cow's milk, but the fat and calorie contents are quite a bit lower. I encourage mothers to think of nonfat milk as the preferred choice and whole milk as nonfat milk with an extra one and a half pats of butter. If you really are stuck on whole milk, you can have it, but you should use less of the foods allowed in the fat group, such as butter and margarine. You'll notice that I list margarine instead of butter in my menus. That is because margarine is made from vegetable oils and contains no cholesterol. As of January 2006 all margarine lists the *trans*-fat content, making it easy to avoid. Read about *trans*-fat on page 160. Both margarine and butter have the same calories. If you love butter and do not have a cholesterol problem, then feel free to use it as your fat serving. Just stick to the portion sizes I recommend.

CAN I EAT THE SAME FOODS MY FAMILY EATS?

Absolutely. The same meals, fruits, vegetables, rice, bread, and so on that other family members eat should be part of your diet, too. The only foods a breastfeeding mother should avoid are those with lots of caffeine or alcohol. Because a mother's calorie needs increase while she's nursing, even the occasional fried food is allowed. What is most important is that you get enough of the six main food groups to supply you with the nutrition you need.

THE NINE FOOD GROUPS

On the following pages is a detailed list of all the foods within each group. At the beginning of each food group read about the specific nutrition those foods provide. Pay close attention to the minimum number of servings suggested.

Both a minimum and a recommended daily serving are listed with each food group. The recommended daily serving numbers equal a 2,700-calorie balanced menu. The minimum servings add up to only 1,800 calories a day. A breastfeeding mother who does not eat the minimum recommended number of servings from the various groups may not be able to meet all her nutritional needs.

Starch Group

These foods are rich in carbohydrate and low in fat. They are also good sources of thiamine, niacin, and iron. Whole grain foods will be good sources of fiber, bran cereals are good sources of zinc, and enriched grains such as fortified breakfast cereal carry folic acid, a nutrient very important to women.

Each serving will give you roughly 80 calories, 15 grams of carbohydrate, 2 to 3 grams of protein, and a trace of fat.

Recommended daily amount	*12 servings*
Minimum daily amount	*7 servings*

Food	Serving Size
Bread (white, rye, raisin, whole wheat, pumpernickel)	1 slice
English muffin, pita bread; hamburger, hot dog, or sandwich roll	½
Tortilla	1
Cereal (flake type, unsweetened)	¾ cup
Cereal (Grape-Nuts, wheat germ, bran concentrate)	⅓ cup
Cereal (uncooked oatmeal or farina)	½ cup

Grains—rice (brown, white, instant), bulgur, grits, pasta, noodles	⅓ cup uncooked
Beans and peas (lentils, kidney, split, black-eyed, lima)	⅓ cup uncooked
Corn	½ cup or 1 ear
Potato (white, sweet)	⅓ cup mashed or 1 small
Winter squash (acorn, butternut)	½ small
Crackers/snacks	
Breadsticks	2 4–inch sticks
Animal crackers	8
Graham crackers	2
Popcorn	3 cups
Crisp crackers (melba toast, pretzels, Ry-Krisp, saltines, nonfat whole wheat)	3–6
Angel cake	1 ½-inch slice
Gingersnaps	3
Bagel	¼

The following are starchy foods that also contain about 5 grams of fat. Eating one serving of these is like eating a starch and a fat; in other words, a slice of bread with butter on it. If you choose these foods, try to cut back on the number of fat servings you eat at the meal.

Popover, scone, doughnut, biscuit, corn bread, muffin, waffle, pancake, coffee cake	1 small serving
Chow mein noodles or fried rice	½ cup
Crackers with fat added	4–6
Taco shells	2

French fries	10
Home fries	½ cup
Cupcake (unfrosted)	1
Plain cake (unfrosted)	1 small serving
Cookie	1 3-inch round
Granola-type cereal	¼ cup

Whole Grains

Whole grains include brown rice, cracked wheat, oatmeal, popcorn, whole barley, whole cornmeal, whole rye, and whole wheat. Foods containing whole grains include bread, crackers, pasta, and cereal. Look for the word *whole* on the ingredients list and compare fiber content on the label to ensure you are getting the real thing. The ongoing Nurses Health Study has found that women who eat three servings of whole grain food each day have less risk of heart disease. Whole grains also protect against diabetes and cancer and they improve digestion. Start the day with a whole grain cereal or toast and have a sandwich on whole wheat bread at lunch and you have met the recommended three servings.

What Is the Glycemic Index?

When a food is eaten, the impact on blood sugar is measured and the glycemic index (GI) is determined for that particular food item (sugar has a GI of 100, brown rice 50, and instant rice 87). Many people oversimplify the GI role in weight control, believing all high-GI foods add to weight gain while foods with a low GI do not. This has led some popular diet books to label foods with a higher GI like kiwi (53) and watermelon (72) to be detrimental to weight loss. But when researchers Alfenas and Mattes fed healthy adults only low-GI foods or only high-GI foods, there were no significant differences in weight gain in either group. This means that the GI content of food is not useful as a meal-planning tool. The glycemic load (GL) is another tool used in diet books and is determined by multiplying a food's GI by the carbohydrate content in the food. The GL is also used by researchers, but it, too, has little practical application for the home cook and menu planner. I include it here because so many people ask about it.

Glycemic Index and Glycemic Load of Selected Foods

Food	GI	GL
Glucose	100	
Cornflakes	92	24
Oatmeal	42	9
Brown rice	50	16
Instant white rice	87	36
White bread	70	10
Whole wheat bread	77	9
Carrots	47	3
Potato	57	12
Apple	38	6
Banana	51	13
Kiwi	53	6
Watermelon	72	4
Whole milk	27	3
Skim milk	32	4

Milk Group

The foods listed below provide approximately 90 calories, 12 grams of carbohydrate, 8 grams of protein, and just a trace of fat per serving. They are also a rich source of vitamin D, riboflavin, and calcium. Nonfat and low-fat milks are encouraged over whole milk because they are equal in nutrition but have many fewer fat calories.

Recommended daily amount	*4 servings*
Minimum daily amount	*3 servings*

Food	Serving Size
Nonfat, ½ percent, 1 percent milk	1 cup
Dry nonfat milk	⅓ cup
Evaporated nonfat milk	½ cup
Low-fat buttermilk	1 cup
Plain, nonfat yogurt	1 cup

Not all mothers drink the milks listed above, so the following foods can be used as additional or substitute sources of calcium. Note how the calorie, protein, and fat composition of these foods differ.

Food	Calories	Carbohydrate (g)	Protein (g)	Fat (g)	Calcium (g)
Skim milk, 1 cup	90	12	8	trace	300
Tofu, 8 ounces	172	6	18	10	308
Collards, 1 cup cooked	51	9.5	5	1	299
Kale, 1½ cups cooked	65	10	8	2	310
Turnip greens, 1 cup cooked	29	5	3	0.3	267
Beet greens, 2 cups cooked	52	10	5	0.6	288
Spinach, 2 cups cooked	82	13	11	1	330
Fruit yogurt, 1 cup	225	42	9	3	314

Goat's milk, 1 cup	168	11	9	10	326
Kefir, 1 cup	160	9	9	5	350
Chocolate milk, 1 percent, 1 cup	160	26	8	3	287
Soy milk, 1 cup calcium fortified	79	4	7	5	300

Calcium and Weight Loss

A study that compared weight loss results of people on high- and low-calcium diets found that people who ate three servings of calcium-rich food daily lost more weight than people who ate only one serving of calcium-rich food or took a supplement. Critics say the study had too few participants to really offer us guidance. Adding low-fat yogurt or skim milk to a diet low in calcium is certainly recommended. These foods are high in nutrients and, unlike salty snack foods, are most unlikely to be eaten in excess. If you already eat the three to four calcium servings suggested here, adding more is not likely to help you lose weight faster.

Protein Group

One serving of each food listed below will contain approximately 7 grams of protein, 3 to 5 grams of fat, and 55 to 75 calories. These protein foods are also good sources of iron, zinc, and thiamine.

Recommended daily amount	*9 servings*
Minimum daily amount	*7 servings*

Food	*Serving Size*
Meat (beef, veal, pork, venison, rabbit, liver, organ meats, poultry without skin, fish)	1 ounce

Canned fish in water (tuna, salmon, crab)	¼ cup
Oysters	6
Cottage cheese, ricotta cheese	¼ cup
Parmesan cheese	2 tablespoons
Mozzarella, low-fat cheeses	1 ounce
Lunch meats, low calorie	1 ounce
Egg	1
Egg substitute	¼ cup
Tofu	4 ounces
Beans (great northern, navy, kidney, lima, black-eyed peas)	½ cup cooked
Baked beans with pork and sweeteners*	½ cup

* Baked beans contain about 8 grams of protein in a ½-cup portion, but the 175 calories per portion is significantly higher than the 75 calories per serving for other foods in this list. Beans can count as a protein or starch serving.

These protein foods are higher in fat and calories. Try to use them less frequently

Cheese, regular	1 ounce
Sausage	1 ounce
Cold cuts	1 ounce
Hot dog	1
Nut butters	1 tablespoon

Nuts

Eating one ounce of nuts four to five times per week significantly reduces a woman's risk of heart disease, and men who eat nuts can lower their cholesterol. The best nuts are walnuts and sunflower seeds because they have the healthiest balance of fat. Almonds, hazelnuts, peanuts, pecans, pine nuts, and pistachio nuts are terrific, too, but there is a catch. To control calories and weight most women should eat their nuts in a meal and not as a snack. Nuts carry about 200 calories in ¼ cup and 5 grams of protein. Eating a peanut butter sandwich instead of a hamburger or adding nuts in a salad instead of cheese is a great way to use them in meals. You will get the health benefits without adding many calories. If you do snack on nuts, control your portion: eating one cup of nuts at 800 calories is far more "fattening" than one cup of blueberries at 100 calories.

Fish Safety

There is a lot of concern about mercury and PCB contamination in fish. Read about fish safety in chapter 8.

Vegetable Group

The foods in this group provide approximately 25 calories per serving. They also contain 5 grams of carbohydrate and 2 grams of protein. They are a good source of vitamin A and vitamin C as well as fiber. Choose a dark green leafy or orange vegetable three or four times a week.

Recommended daily amount   *5 servings*
Minimum daily amount   *4 servings*

A serving is ½ cup cooked vegetable or juice or 1 cup raw vegetable.

Food

Asparagus	Mushrooms
Bean sprouts	Okra
Beans, green and wax	Onions
Beets	Pea pods
Broccoli	Peppers, all colors
Brussels sprouts	Rutabaga
Cabbage	Sauerkraut

Carrot juice   Spinach
Carrots   Tomatoes
Cauliflower   Tomato juice
Eggplant   Turnips
Greens   Yellow squash
Kohlrabi   Zucchini
Leeks

Starchy vegetables such as peas, corn, and potatoes are listed under the starch group.

Fruit Group

Each serving provides approximately 70 calories and 15 grams of carbohydrate. These foods are a rich source of fiber and vitamin C.

Recommended daily amount	*6 servings*
Minimum daily amount	*4 servings*

Food	Serving Size
Apple, kiwi, nectarine, orange, peach, pear	1 whole
Plums, persimmons, tangerines, apricots, figs	2 small
Berries	1 cup
Melon cubes	1 cup
Juice (apple, grapefruit, orange, pineapple)	½ cup
Juice (cranberry, grape, prune, cherry)	⅓ cup
Applesauce, fruit cocktail	½ cup
Banana	½ large or 1 small
Cherries	12
Grapes	15
Mango	¾ cup or ½ large

Pineapple, canned	⅓ cup
Pomegranate	½
Dried fruit	
Apples	4 rings
Apricots	7 halves
Dates	2
Figs	2
Prunes	3
Raisins	2 tablespoons

Choose Whole Fruit Over Juice or Dried Fruit

Whole fruit makes an ideal snack but juice and dried fruit can be problems. Even though it carries more nutrients, juice has the same calories as soft drinks. Dried fruit can be problematic when trying to cut calories because all the water has been removed; water in whole grapes makes people feel full, but when served in the form of raisins, the absence of water might not make you feel full. Some people eat dried fruit like candy, consuming a lot more calories than one would expect if eating whole grapes.

Fat Group

These foods contain approximately 5 grams of fat and 45 calories per serving. Foods that come from animal sources contain cholesterol and saturated fat and tend to raise blood cholesterol levels. The best fats to choose are those that carry little saturated fat and no *trans*-fat: soft margarine, salad dressings made with canola oil and olive oil. Read labels to compare fat content.

Recommended daily amount	*7 servings*
Minimum daily amount	*5 servings*

Food	*Serving Size*
Margarine, mayonnaise, all cooking oils, butter	1 teaspoon

Diet margarine, diet mayonnaise, mayonnaise-type salad dressing	1 tablespoon
Salad dressing, oil variety	1 tablespoon
Diet salad dressing	2 tablespoons
Olives	10 small, 5 large
Nuts	
Peanuts	10 large, 20 small
Cashews, pine nuts, sunflower seeds	1 tablespoon
Almonds, dry roasted	6
Cream	
Heavy	1 tablespoon
Light	2 tablespoons
Sour	2 tablespoons
Cream cheese	1 tablespoon
Coffee whitener, liquid	2 tablespoons
Coffee whitener, powder	1 tablespoon
Gravy, homemade or canned	1 tablespoon

Free Foods Group

These foods are so low in calories that they don't need to be considered in your total food intake, but in most cases they don't have much nutritional value, either. Sugar-free products are listed here, but I rarely encourage the use of sugar substitutes or the products that have them. I only recommend them if a person has diabetes. All breastfeeding mothers can afford the 10 to 20 calories in a teaspoon of sugar, honey, or jam—so enjoy the real thing.

Food
Bouillon
Carbonated drinks, diet
Carbonated water and club soda with fruit flavors

Cocoa powder, unsweetened
Coffee or tea (Limit all coffee to 2 cups a day, black tea to 2 to
    3 cups. Herbal tea is caffeine free and can be enjoyed in rea-
    sonable quantities.)
Drink mixes, sugar free
Tonic water, sugar free
Nonstick pan spray
Fruit
    Cranberries, raw
    Rhubarb, raw
Vegetables
    Celery
    Chinese cabbage
    Cucumbers
    Green onions
    Hot peppers
    Radishes
Salad Greens
    Endive
    Escarole
    Lettuce
    Romaine
Candy, hard, sugar free
Gelatin, sugar free
Gum, sugar free
Jam or jelly, sugar free
Sugar substitutes such as saccharin or aspartame
Whipped topping, 2 tablespoons
Condiments
    Catsup
    Horseradish
    Mustard
    Pickles, dill, unsweetened
    Taco sauce
    Vinegar

Seasonings
    Dry or fresh herbs and spices
    Flavoring extracts (almond, butter, lemon, peppermint,
        vanilla, walnut, etc.)
    Hot pepper sauce
    Lemon
    Lemon juice
    Lime
    Lime juice
    Soy sauce
    Wine used in cooking
    Worcestershire sauce

Combination Food Group

Much of the food we eat is mixed together in various combinations that don't fit easily into only one food group. It can be quite hard to tell what is in a certain casserole or baked food. The list below explains the food groups for some typical combination foods.

Food	Food Groups
Meat and cheese casseroles, made with noodles, rice, or potato, 1 cup	1 starch, 2 vegetable, 2 protein
Cheese pizza, 2 small slices	2 starch, 1 protein, 1 fat
Chili with beans, 1 cup	2 starch, 2 meat, 2 fat
Chow mein without noodles or rice, 2 cups	1 starch, 2 vegetable, 2 protein
Macaroni and cheese, 1 cup	2 starch, 1 protein, 2 fat
Soups	
Bean, 1 cup	1 starch, 1 vegetable, 1 protein
Chunky, all varieties, 1 10¾-ounce can	1 starch, 1 vegetable, 1 protein
Cream, canned, made with water, 1 cup	1 starch, 1 fat

Vegetable, without potatoes or corn, 1 cup	1 vegetable
Vegetable, with potatoes or corn, 1 cup	1 starch

Sugar-free pudding made with nonfat milk, ½ cup	1 starch

Daily Option Group

These foods don't really fit into any category, but they taste good and a nursing mother can certainly enjoy them. They provide calories but very little nutrition. Try to use only one of these foods a day. One serving provides about 50 calories. The sugar-free alternatives can be used, but since I don't encourage the use of artificial sweeteners (unless a mother is diabetic), I'd rather see you enjoy the real thing. Read more about sugar substitutes on page 111.

Food	Serving Size
Maple syrup	1 tablespoon
Jam or jelly	1 tablespoon
Life Savers	6 pieces
Regular soda	6 ounces
White or brown sugar	1 tablespoon
Honey	1 tablespoon
Chocolate candy	½ ounce
Chocolate syrup	1 tablespoon

You can follow the following sample exactly or use the food groups given as a good reference for designing your own menu. If you wish, you can mix and match breakfasts, lunches, and suppers from different days. Water, coffee, and tea are free foods, and you can include them at any meal (but first, read about coffee in chapter 8). Recipes for foods marked with an asterisk are included in chapter 10.

Tips on Losing Weight While Breastfeeding

- Don't skip breakfast—even a small yogurt is better than nothing.
- Eat three meals and include some protein and at least three other food items. A sandwich made with two slices of bread, chicken, lettuce, and tomato or a vegetable soup with a glass of milk, bread, and butter are examples. Protein can come from the meat group or the milk group.
- When hungry between meals, choose food from the milk, fruit, or vegetable group, or select one serving from the starch group.
- Don't get too hungry. Hunger can lead to overeating. Being a little hungry before meals is perfect. Feeling so hungry you eat a whole bag of chips uncontrollably is obviously a problem.

A Week's Menu for Breastfeeding Mothers

DAY ONE

Food	Exchanges
Breakfast	
½–1 cup fruit juice	1–2 fruit
¾ cup bran flakes	1 starch
½–1 cup skim milk	½–1 milk
1 English muffin with 1–2 teaspoons margarine	2 starch, 1–2 fat
Snack	
½ cup plain yogurt with 1 tablespoon honey or syrup	½ milk, 1 daily option
3–6 graham crackers	1–2 starch
Lunch	
Quick-Cooking Chili,* 1 ¾-cup portion	3 protein, 2 starch, 2 vegetable, 1 fat

1 cup salad with 1 tablespoon dressing	1 vegetable, 1 fat
1 cup skim milk	1 milk

Snack

1 slice cheese melted on ½ pita bread with chopped tomato	1 protein, 1 starch, 1 vegetable
½ cup fruit juice or apple	1 fruit

Supper

4 ounces salmon, broiled	4 protein
1 cup skim milk	1 milk
½–1 cup steamed carrots with 1 teaspoon margarine	1–2 vegetable, 1 fat
1 baked potato	1 starch
1 cup salad with 1 tablespoon dressing	1 vegetable, 1 fat
1 small ear of corn with 1 teaspoon margarine	1 starch, 1 fat
Small bunch of grapes	1 fruit

Snack

½ cup skim milk	½ milk
¾–1½ cups cereal	1–2 starch
½ banana	1 fruit

DAY TWO

Food	Exchanges

Breakfast

Two-egg vegetable omelet (Melt 1 teaspoon margarine in omelet pan, add 2 beaten eggs. Let set a bit. Sprinkle with ½ cup of mixed vegetables; try tomato, mushroom, and onion. Cook until done.)	2 protein, 1 fat, 1 vegetable

| 1 English muffin with 1 teaspoon margarine | 2 starch, 1 fat |
| ½–1 cup orange juice | 1–2 fruit |

Snack

| Yogurt shake (1 cup plain yogurt blended with 1 cup strawberries) | 1 milk, 1 fruit |
| 1–2 slices raisin toast with 1 teaspoon margarine | 1–2 starch, 1 fat |

Lunch

Crab salad sandwich (3 ounces crabmeat, canned or fresh, 1 tablespoon diet mayonnaise, and chopped celery or onion on a whole wheat roll)	2 starch, 3 protein, 1 fat
½–1 cup Broccoli Salad*	1–2 vegetable, 1 fat
½–1 cup skim milk	½–1 milk

Snack

½ banana	1 fruit
2 rice cakes	1 starch
½ cup skim milk	½ milk

Supper

4 ounces Vegetable Meat Loaf*	4 protein, 1 vegetable, 1 starch
1–2 small oven-roasted potatoes	1–2 starch
½ cup green beans with 1 teaspoon margarine	1 vegetable, 1 fat
1¼ strawberries	1 fruit
1 cup skim milk	1 milk

Snack

| ½ bagel with 1 tablespoon cream cheese | 2 starch, 1 fat |
| ½ cup skim milk | ½ milk |

DAY THREE

Food	Exchanges

Breakfast

Food	Exchanges
½ grapefruit	1 fruit
1 cup yogurt with 3 tablespoons wheat germ and 10 sliced grapes	1 milk, 1 starch, 1 fruit
1–2 slices toast with 1–2 teaspoons margarine	1–2 starch, 1–2 fat
½ cup skim milk	½ milk
1 tablespoon peanut butter on 1 slice toast	1 protein, 1 starch

Lunch

Food	Exchanges
Tuna sandwich (½ cup tuna with 2 teaspoons mayonnaise on 2 slices toast with sliced tomato)	2 protein, 2 fat, 2 starch, 1 vegetable
1 cup carrot and cucumber sticks with diet dressing	1 vegetable, 1 fat
1 cup skim milk	1 milk
1 apple	1 fruit

Snack

Food	Exchanges
¼ cup cottage cheese on ½ bagel with sliced tomato	1 protein, 2 starch, 1 vegetable
½–1 cup fruit juice	1–2 fruit

Supper

Food	Exchanges
3 Salmon Croquettes*	4 protein, 1 starch, 1 fat
½ cup Yogurt Dill Sauce*	½ milk
½–1 cup steamed carrots	1–2 vegetable
½–1 cup cooked rice with 1 teaspoon margarine	1–2 starch, 1 fat
Baked Pear*	1 fruit, 1 daily option
½ cup skim milk	½ milk

Snack

½ cup skim milk	½ milk
3 cups salted air-popped popcorn	1 starch

DAY FOUR

Food	Exchanges

Breakfast

· 2–3 slices French toast (2–3 slices whole wheat bread dipped in 2 eggs scrambled with ½ cup milk. Cook in 1–2 teaspoons of margarine until done. Sprinkle with nutmeg.)	2–3 starch, 2 protein, ½ milk, 1–2 fat
Top with ½ cup yogurt and 1 cup Blueberry Sauce*	option
½ cup orange juice	1 fruit

Snack

3 graham crackers	1 starch
¾ cup skim milk	¾ milk

Lunch

1 cup vegetable soup	1 vegetable
1 pita filled with Curried Chicken*	3 protein, 1 fat, ¼ milk, 1 fruit, 2 starch
½–1 cup Broccoli Salad*	1–2 vegetable, 1 fat

Snack

3 graham crackers	1 starch
½–1 cup fruit juice	1–2 fruit

Supper

1 cup skim milk	1 milk
3 ounces marinated steak	3 meat

½–1 cup mashed potato with 1 tablespoon gravy	1–2 starch, 1 fat
½ cup corn kernels with 1 tablespoon margarine	1 starch, 1 fat
½–1 cup green beans with 1 teaspoon margarine	1–2 vegetables, 1 fat
1 slice angel cake with strawberries	1 starch, 1 fruit

Snack

½ cup skim milk	½ milk
8 animal crackers	1 starch

DAY FIVE

Food	Exchanges

Breakfast

1 cup skim milk	1 milk
¾–1 ½ cups bran flakes with ½ banana, sliced	1–2 starch, 1 fruit
1 slice toast with 1 tablespoon peanut butter	1 starch, 1 protein
½–1 cup orange juice	1–2 fruit

Snack

½ cup skim milk	½ milk
3 graham crackers	1 starch

Lunch

Mexican salad sandwich (Sauté 2 ounces ground turkey in 1 teaspoon vegetable oil and ¼ cup salsa. Divide between two warmed soft flour tortillas. Top with 1 ounce grated cheese, shredded lettuce, and tomato.)	3 protein, 2 starch, 1–2 vegetable, 1 fat

1 cup skim milk	1 milk
1 apple	1 fruit

Snack

½ cup apple juice	1 fruit
½ bagel with 1 tablespoon cream cheese	2 starch, 1 fat
½ cup milk	½ milk

Supper

2 pieces Yogurt-Fried Chicken*	4 protein, ½ milk, 1 starch
½–1 cup cooked carrots and green beans with 2 teaspoons margarine	1–2 vegetable, 2 fat
1 cup salad with 1 tablespoon dressing and 1 tablespoon sunflower seeds	1 vegetable, 2 fat
½–1 cup cooked rice with 1 teaspoon margarine	1–2 starch, 1 fat
⅓ cantaloupe	1 fruit

Snack

½ cup skim milk	½ milk
2–4 breadsticks	1–2 starch

DAY SIX

Food	Exchanges

Breakfast

2 slices raisin toast with 1–2 teaspoons margarine	2 starch, 1–2 fat
1 cup yogurt with ½ cup fruit and 3 tablespoons wheat germ	1 milk, 1 fruit, 1 starch
½–1 cup orange juice	1–2 fruit
1 ounce turkey sausage	1 protein

Snack

½ cup yogurt with 3 tablespoons wheat germ and 1 tablespoon honey	½ milk, 1 starch, 1 daily option
½ banana	1 fruit

Lunch

Brown Rice and Broccoli*	2 starch, 3 protein, 2 vegetable, 1 fat
1 orange	1 fruit
1 cup skim milk	1 milk

Snack

1 hard-cooked egg with 1–2 teaspoons mayonnaise on 1–2 slices toast with sliced tomato	1 protein, 1–2 fat, 1–2 starch, 1 vegetable

Supper

3 ounces roast turkey	3 protein
½–1 cup stuffing with 2 tablespoons gravy	1–2 starch, 1 fat
½–1 cup steamed broccoli and carrots with 1 teaspoon margarine	1–2 vegetable, 1 fat
¼ cup sherbet with ½ cup sliced peaches	1 starch, 1 fruit
1 cup skim milk	1 milk

Snack

½ cup skim milk	½ milk
3 graham crackers	1 starch

DAY SEVEN

Food	Exchange

Breakfast

Food	Exchange
1 English muffin with 1–2 teaspoons margarine	2 starch, 1–2 fat
1 cup skim milk with ¾ cup cereal	1 milk, 1 starch
½ banana	1 fruit
½–1 cup orange juice	1–2 fruit

Snack

Food	Exchange
½ cup skim milk	½ milk
3 gingersnaps	1 starch

Lunch

Food	Exchange
3 ounces lean cold cuts on a roll with 1–2 teaspoons mayonnaise	3 protein, 2 starch, 1–2 fat
1 cup skim milk	1 milk
1 cup sliced tomato and cucumber salad with 1 tablespoon French dressing	1 vegetable, 1 fat

Snack

Food	Exchange
1 ounce sliced cheese on ½ cup apple or pear slices	1 protein, 1 fruit
½ cup skim milk pudding	1 milk

Supper

Food	Exchange
1 cup skim milk	1 milk
1 cup Quick Spaghetti Sauce* over 1–1½ cups pasta	2–3 starch
1 cup salad with 2 tablespoons diet dressing	1 vegetable, 1 fat
1 cup cooked zucchini with 1 teaspoon margarine	2 vegetable, 1 fat
½ cup apple juice	1 fruit

Snack

Fruit frappe (½ cup plain yogurt
   blended with ¼ cup sherbet or
   frozen yogurt and ½ banana or
   1 cup frozen strawberries)   ½ milk, 1 starch, 1 fruit

* Recipe provided in chapter 10.

CAN I SNACK AT NIGHT?

Many mothers look forward to a special snack once the children
are put to bed. This is a time to put your feet up, have an undis-
turbed conversation, or just savor the taste of a yogurt sundae in
peace. Of course, the best choices are those in the seven-day
menu. However, if chocolate cake, ice cream, or cookies are calling you, my advice is to take a portion, put it on a plate or in a
bowl, sit down, and really enjoy it. Most "snackers" get into
trouble when they eat mindlessly—standing in front of the refrigerator, grabbing food on the way through the kitchen, or eating the leftovers on a dinner plate. The most important thing
you can do to manage what you eat is to manage how you eat.
You can do this by being mindful; sit down and really enjoy what
you chose.

THIS IS WAY TOO MUCH FOOD

If the portions on the menu seem too large, reduce the starch and
fat servings. Don't eliminate the fruits or vegetables—they prevent disease and you need to get into the habit of including them
at every meal so you control your weight permanently and so
you set a good example for your children. Always include a food
that carries some protein (foods from the meat or milk group).

WHAT IF I DON'T EAT THE FOODS
ON THE MENU?

Menu plans can't match the likes and dislikes of everyone who uses them. That's the beauty of the food-group system. If I recommend three starches at breakfast, it doesn't matter if you eat three slices of toast or three waffles or a cup and a half of oatmeal. All three foods are similar in nutritional value and calories. You can choose the food you like. What I don't recommend is switching from one food group to another, eating fewer servings, or skipping meals or snacks altogether.

YOUR MENU LASTS FOR ONLY ONE WEEK—
WHAT DO I DO AFTER THAT?

Use this menu as a guide. It's meant to be enlightening, not enslaving, so please don't feel you must be ruled by it. It can help you learn about how much food you need and which foods will help provide the nutrients you need. Even if you plan to follow my menu exactly, you'll soon find that rigidity won't always work. Special occasions do come up: A friend drops by with sub sandwiches and your menu says crabmeat salad. Or maybe your mother babysits for an evening so you can treat yourself to a much-deserved dinner out. Try to be flexible.

HOW WILL I KNOW IF I'M GETTING
ENOUGH TO EAT?

If you're hungry all the time or are losing more than one pound per week, you're probably not eating enough. To help with hunger, get enough lean protein and include some high-fiber foods such as fruits or vegetables because the fiber helps with satiety. The best way I know to evaluate your food intake is to keep a food diary. Write down what you eat and the groups the foods represent, and compare your list to the servings I have recommended from each food group. If you aren't eating the minimum number of servings from any of the groups, you must start eating more. If you have no appetite and can't seem to make yourself eat, talk to your doctor or find a registered dietitian for personalized advice.

I FEEL AS IF I NEED TO EAT MORE AT THE MORNING SNACK—WHAT SHOULD I DO?

Once again, don't be a slave to my menu. It's fine for you to switch the portions around, but try not to go below or above the recommended number of servings from any food group. If you want to add fruit to your morning snack, add it and consider skipping the fruit suggested for the afternoon snack.

HOW TO INDIVIDUALIZE YOUR MENU

Use the worksheet in table 5 to determine your calorie needs more precisely. Using this information, you'll be able to adapt the Natural Diet for Mothers to help you lose weight. But remember, never go below the daily minimum number of servings of any food group while breastfeeding.

Table 5. Estimating Your Calorie Requirements

First, *determine your goal weight (also called ideal body weight, or IBW)*: you can also use prepregnancy weight, weight at age twenty-one, or refer to the BMI on page 222. A BMI between 19 and 25 is a recommended weight goal.

Medium frame	Allow 100 pounds for the first 5 feet of height plus 5 pounds for each additional inch.
Small frame	Subtract 10 percent from total for medium frame.
Large frame	Add 10 percent to total for medium frame.

For example, a medium-frame five-foot, eight-inch woman should weigh 140 pounds.

Your goal weight or IBW is _____.

Then multiply your goal weight by the activity number that matches your exercise habits. Most of us fall in the sedentary category unless we engage in regular exercise. Mothers who exercise twenty to thirty minutes three times a week are engaging in moderate exercise. If you are doing less exercise, count yourself in the sedentary group. If you exercise more often and for a longer duration, then you are probably engaging in heavy exercise.

13 for	Sedentary activity (some walking, typing, sewing, ironing, cooking, seated and standing activities, light housekeeping)
15 for	Moderate activity (walking briskly, weeding, hoeing, carrying loads, bicycling, tennis, dancing)
20 for	Heavy activity (jogging, heavy manual labor, climbing, digging)

Your daily calorie requirement when not breastfeeding (IBW × activity number) is _____.

Finally, add to this total the 330 to 450 calories needed each day to make breast milk.

Your calorie range when breastfeeding is _____.

For example, if your goal weight is 140 pounds and you are usually sedentary, you'd multiply your activity number of 13 by 140 pounds and come up with 1,820 calories. This is the number of calories you'd need if you weren't breastfeeding and wanted to maintain your ideal weight. Since you are breastfeeding, you need to add 330 to 450 calories, for a daily total of 2,150 to 2,270 calories (round it off to 2,200).

Those 2,200 calories should theoretically allow adequate nourishment for you plus just enough to ensure an adequate supply of breast milk, while encouraging your body to burn some of the fat you stored while pregnant.

WHAT IF I WAS UNDERWEIGHT WHEN I DELIVERED MY BABY?

If you didn't gain enough weight while pregnant, you'll want to eat 500 to 650 extra calories. This amount should keep you from losing any more weight. To gain weight, you may need to eat even more, perhaps a total of 3,000 calories a day.

CALORIES AREN'T THE WHOLE STORY

Calories are important, but there's more to losing weight safely. After all, a mother could eat 2,300 calories of ice cream every day and lose weight, but she'd feel miserable because her intake of essential nutrients would be inadequate. Also be mindful of your weight loss. If you are losing more than one pound per week, your calorie intake is probably too low.

Use your calorie needs as the starting point for planning a good, healthy diet. Nutritionists now recommend that we break up our calorie intake as follows:

Protein = 20 percent of total calories, or a bit less
Carbohydrate = 50 percent of total calories, or up to 60 percent
Fat = 25 to 35 percent of total calories

These percentages will affect your food choices differently at different calorie levels (see table 6). Round your expected daily calorie level off to the nearest hundred and find how many servings of each food group you should choose each day.

What About Low-Carbohydrate Diets While Breastfeeding?

Researchers Doberne and Heinig set out to answer the question: What do we know about low-carbohydrate diets while breastfeeding? The answer was virtually nothing. According to the researchers, the diets are hard to stick to and they may impact breast milk production. It is estimated that breastfeeding mothers need 210 grams of carbohydrate to meet their brain's requirement for energy and to replace the carbohydrate used in making breast milk. A low-carb diet may provide only 50 to 60 grams of carbohydrate for the whole day, potentially causing ketosis, a condition in which the body exclusively relies on stored fat for energy instead of carbohydrate. As a result, chemicals called ketones build up in the blood. Ketones impact the taste and smell of milk, making it less desirable and potentially decreasing your baby's intake. Not only could a low-carbohydrate diet impact your nursing experience, it is not even guaranteed to help with long-term weight loss. When researchers looked at the efficacy of losing weight on a low-carbohydrate diet, they had to conclude that there was "insufficient evidence for or against the use of low-carbohydrate diets." The weight loss that occurs while on a low-carbohydrate diet actually is the result of reduced calorie intake, not less carbohydrate. A menu low in carbohydrate can cause rapid weight loss because the body releases water when carbohydrate is restricted. But when researchers assessed the weight lost in men and women weighing an average of 288 pounds, they found a loss of 12 pounds over six months. Twelve pounds is significant, but not the amount most dieters expect when they hear all the hype associated with these diets.

Your body needs carbohydrate while breastfeeding. Do not turn to a restrictive diet while nursing. It might compromise your milk production and it might not even be very effective.

Table 6. Food Choices for a Balanced Menu

Daily Calories   *Servings*

	Milk (skim)	Meat	Starch	Vegetable	Fruit	Fat
1,800	3	7	7	4	4	5
1,900	3	7	8	4	4	5
2,000	3	7	9	4	4	6
2,100	3	7	9	4	5	6
2,200	3	7	10	4	5	7
2,300	3	7	10	4	6	7
2,400	4	8	10	4	6	7
2,500	4	8	11	4	6	7
2,600	4	8	11	5	6	7
2,700	4	8	12	5	6	7
2,800	4	9	12	6	6	8
2,900	4	9	13	6	6	9
3,000	4	9	13	7	6	10

Caution: At less than 2,300 calories a day, your intake of calcium may be low because you're only getting three milk servings. To ensure adequate calcium, choose at least one good alternate vegetable calcium source, such as a healthy serving of green leafy vegetables, or choose cheese, tofu, or canned fish with bones as one of your protein selections.

At 2,200 calories and below mothers must make very good food selections to meet all their nutrient needs. They may have a difficult time getting calcium, zinc, vitamin B_6, folic acid, magnesium, thiamine, iron, selenium, vitamin E, riboflavin, and niacin. Mothers eating near or at the 1,800-calorie level will need a multivitamin (read about supplements in chapter 2).

To adjust the week's menu to meet the calorie level you have calculated for yourself, simply compare the servings listed for your new calorie level to those on the seven-day sample menu and adjust accordingly. Eating the greatest portions on the sample menu will add up to 2,700 calories; a mother needing 2,500 calories a day could eat one less starch serving and one less serving from the vegetable group.

HOW OFTEN SHOULD I CHECK MY WEIGHT?

Check it only if you feel the need to and no more than once a week, preferably first thing in the morning on the same day of each week. Try not to let the scale be your only guide to good health. I recommend that you focus attention on eating good food and getting regular, gentle exercise. If you are able to combine these two, then the scale will start to head in the direction you want.

CAN I HAVE SUGAR?

Sugar contains about 15 calories per teaspoon. It provides no nutrition, but if used in small amounts, I don't believe it does any harm. Personally, I prefer the taste of honey as a sweetener, but neither honey nor sugar can be called nutritious.

Honey and sugar are part of my daily option group. One serving of these foods a day is fine.

Sugar Substitutes

What to choose when you want to satisfy your sweet tooth? The Center for Science in the Public Interest (CSPI) recently reviewed the nonnutritive sugar replacements and made these conclusions. The full article can be read at their website, listed below.

- Sucralose, also called Splenda, "has passed all safety tests."
- Neotame, a combination of the same ingredients used to make aspartame. "Unlike aspartame, neotame is not broken down in the body into the amino acid phenylalanine, which is toxic to people with phenylketonuria (PKU). Animal and human studies have raised no safety concerns."
- Sugar alcohols: erythritol, hydrogenated starch hydrolysates (polyglycitol, polyglucitol), isomalt, lactitol, maltitol, mannitol, sorbitol, and xylitol. Sugar alcohols are considered "safe" but may cause diarrhea when consumed in large amounts.
- Tagatose, also called Naturlose. Made from milk sugar, most of it passes through the body unabsorbed. Because it is not absorbed, it can cause gas, bloating, flatulence, and nausea. Considered "safe," though it may cause gastrointestinal problems.
- Aspartame, also known as Equal, NutraSweet, and Natra Taste. Aspartame consumed in moderation is "probably safe." However, Dr. Ruth Lawrence writes in her textbook *Breastfeeding: A Guide for the Medical Profession* that breastfeeding women are advised to limit aspartame's use because it can increase phenylalanine in breast milk.
- Acesulfame, also called Sweet One, Sunett, acesulfame potassium. It is a synthetic chemical our bodies cannot metabolize and until better tested, CSPI suggests it be avoided.
- Stevia, also called Sweet Leaf and Honey Leaf, is extracted from a shrub and cannot be metabolized by the human body. The CSPI states that tests have been inadequate.
- Saccharin, also called Sweet'N Low, is considered unsafe.

Source: www.cspinet.org/nah/05_04/sweet_nothings.pdf.

DOES A WOMAN WITH A BIGGER BABY NEED TO EAT MORE FOOD THAN I DO?

Babies need to eat about 45 calories a day per pound, so a baby weighing three pounds more than yours needs an extra 135 calories a day. If both babies are exclusively breastfed, the bigger baby will need to eat that extra food from her mom's breast milk, and her mother will need to eat more than you to provide it. If the larger baby is more than six months old, she can get her extra calories from eating solids (preferably iron-rich foods) instead of from her mom.

SHOULD I EAT LESS WHEN MY BABY STARTS TO EAT SOLIDS?

By the time she's six months old, a baby can start on solid foods. In fact, a baby should start on solids then because she needs the nutrients, such as iron, that supplemental foods provide. There is no exact way to determine your calorie needs when your baby is nursing and eating solids. I suggest you let your appetite and body weight guide you. If you aren't hungry between meals, then you're probably getting all the food you need. If you're losing more than one pound a week, then you probably need to eat more. If you have reached your ideal weight, you want to eat enough to prevent further weight loss.

I DON'T WANT TO LOSE ANY MORE WEIGHT BUT I CAN'T STOP!

Some women can't keep weight on while breastfeeding. Frequent snacking and three good sit-down meals can help. You should also keep a food record and evaluate whether you're getting all the servings you need from the recommended food groups. If not, add the ones you're missing. Make sure you get protein at every meal and one or two servings from the fat group such as margarine, mayonnaise, or salad dressing. If you are getting the amounts you thought you needed but you're still losing, then add an extra 200 calories per day by adding two starches and one extra serving of lean meat, or an extra cup of low-fat milk and one starch serving. Nuts make a great snack for women wanting to gain weight: they contain fiber, protein, healthy fat, and 200 calories in ¼ cup.

WHAT IF I NEED MORE HELP WITH MY DIET?

Nothing beats sitting down with a registered dietitian or a lactation consultant who has training in nutrition for personal guidance. But you can do a good job of evaluating your own diet by keeping a food diary. If you don't have time, a checklist like the one shown in table 7 can do just as well. Each time you eat a food, check off the food group it belongs in. Use one check for each serving you consume.

Table 7. Food Checklist

Each time you eat, check off the food groups consumed, one check for each food-exchange portion. For example, if you eat two slices of toast with two teaspoons of margarine at 7:00 A.M., you should place two checks in the starch box and two in the fat box in the 6:00 A.M.–10:00 A.M. time slot. If you eat a combination food, check all the food groups that make up the dish. For example, 1½ cups of a casserole may merit two checks in the starch group, one in the protein, and one in the fat category. Free foods don't need to be marked, but put one check at the bottom of the page for each daily option food consumed.

Exchange Portions Eaten

6:00 A.M.–10:00 A.M.
Protein _____
Starch _____
Milk _____
Fruit _____
Vegetable _____
Fat _____

10:00 A.M.–2:00 P.M.
Protein _____
Starch _____
Milk _____
Fruit _____
Vegetable _____
Fat _____

2:00 P.M.–6:00 P.M.
Protein _____
Starch _____
Milk _____
Fruit _____
Vegetable _____
Fat _____

6:00 P.M.–10:00 P.M.
Protein _____
Starch _____
Milk _____
Fruit _____
Vegetable _____
Fat _____

10:00 P.M.–6:00 A.M.

Protein   _____

Starch   _____

Milk _____

Fruit   _____

Vegetable _____

Fat _____

Daily Option   _____

Now add up the checks in each category, enter them below, and compare your actual intake of each food group with the servings recommended in table 6:

	Actual Intake	*Recommended Intake*
Protein	_____	_____
Starch	_____	_____
Milk	_____	_____
Fruit	_____	_____
Vegetable	_____	_____
Fat	_____	_____

THE KEY TO YOUR SUCCESS IS STARTING OVER

In my experience, the greatest obstacle to weight loss and improved eating is that we think dieting is an all-or-nothing proposition. We start off highly motivated, but when we stray and eat what we think is inappropriate or "bad," we give up. It's very important to understand that you will never be a "perfect" eater. There will be times when all goes right and other times when you overeat or eat a high-calorie–high-fat food. The key to dietary success is to just start over. So please don't be disappointed in yourself if you don't eat the perfect menu every meal and every day. Just reestablish your goals and start over as often as you need to.

7

EXERCISE—IT'S WORTH IT

Adding exercise to your incredibly busy life may seem impossible (or masochistic), but it's worth doing. A new mother can get some much-needed toning from exercise, along with a wonderful sense of well-being. After all, you take care of the baby, but who's taking care of you?

The benefits of exercise are numerous. It maintains good muscle tone and protects against back pain. A sound exercise program can help prevent heart disease, osteoporosis, and obesity. It even helps with depression. Exercise does more than just burn calories; it actually increases your metabolism. One study found that after a person exercises, her metabolic rate (the speed at which she burns calories) can increase by 10 percent, and it can stay that way for up to forty-eight hours. Instead of making us hungry, exercise usually acts as an appetite controller. *It doesn't really matter what you do. The key to an exercise program is to find something you like and just do it.*

WHEN CAN I START TO EXERCISE?

Only your doctor knows the answer to this since he or she knows your medical condition. If you had an uncomplicated delivery and are in good health, you can probably start right away. A mother who had a cesarean birth may need to wait four weeks or more.

A woman who has recently given birth is in a unique physical state: she suddenly stops balancing the weight of her pregnant abdomen at the same time she undergoes musculoskeletal changes that can leave her a bit unsteady. Add this to the fact that most of us aren't active in those last months of pregnancy, and you can see why you need to take it slow at first. You have a lot of demands on you, and there's no need to overdo it.

BABIES CAN CHANGE OLD EXERCISE HABITS

Once your bundle of joy arrives, finding time for exercise can be much more difficult. If you arrange to have a half hour of time to call your own, you may have to choose between going for a walk, doing the laundry, or taking a much-desired nap.

Before I had children, I could schedule a walk anytime I felt like it. As a result I had no schedule, and at the end of the week my plans for taking three full walks had resulted in only one actual walk. After having Sarah, it was terribly difficult to arrange time for myself. The only way to pull it off was to schedule an appointment with my husband so that he could take care of her. Then when we had two little girls we had to schedule regular exercise periods. As a result, I got more exercise than I usually did.

Be realistic about what you can take on while caring for a new baby. It's great if you can manage to have fun with the baby, have time for yourself, keep the house clean, be involved in the community, work at home or at a job, take care of the rest of your family, and exercise, too. But maybe you can't. Please don't despair. Your baby will grow up sooner than you can imagine, and there will be a time when you will once again be able to plan exercise whenever you wish.

What to Do With the Baby While You Exercise

- Hire a babysitter.
- Arrange to swap exercise time with another mom. She watches your baby while you exercise and you do the same for her.
- Join a gym that offers child care services on the premises.
- Exercise while the baby sleeps.
- Put the baby in a swinging seat and let him watch you while you exercise to a tape or TV.
- Get up early and exercise before the baby wakes up.
- Form a new moms' exercise group at home and have one mom care for the babies while the rest of you work out.

EXERCISE GUIDELINES FOR NEW MOTHERS

Since exercise really is different for new mothers, be careful how you start. The following recommendations are based on guidelines put out by the American College of Obstetricians and Gynecologists (ACOG).

1. Swimming, walking, biking, aerobic dancing, and jogging are all acceptable if performed correctly.
2. Do not exercise vigorously in hot, humid weather or if you have a fever.
3. Avoid jerky, bouncy movements; jumping; jarring motions; or activities that require quick changes in direction. Exercise on a wooden floor or a lightly carpeted floor to reduce chances of injury.
4. Warm up before vigorous activity by walking or bicycling on a stationary bike for five minutes.
5. Cool down for five to twenty minutes after vigorous exercise. Follow with a period of gradually declining activity and stretch to prevent soreness. Because your joints are still somewhat loose after you deliver, don't take stretches to their point of maximum resistance.

6. Check your heart rate by taking your pulse and comparing it to the heart rate guidelines for postpartum mothers listed in the box below. Mothers should not exceed these rates unless they have consulted their doctors.

7. When doing floor exercises, rise from the floor slowly to prevent low blood pressure. Gently exercise your legs following floor exercises.

8. Drink enough fluids to prevent thirst and dehydration.

9. If you were sedentary before you had your baby, begin exercise gradually and advance slowly.

Check Your Pulse

When exercising, checking your pulse will let you know if you are working hard enough to receive health benefits—or if you are working too hard. The chart below lists the target heart rate (THR) for postpartum women while exercising in the second column. The THR is usually 220 minus one's age, and is usually 60 to 80 percent of one's maximum heart rate. The third column lists the maximum number of beats for a sixty-second interval. Take your pulse while exercising. If the number of beats exceeds the recommended amount, you are doing too much and should slow down gradually. If your pulse isn't up to the recommended number, pick up the pace a bit and test your pulse again.

Target Heart Rate General Guidelines for Postpartum Exercise

Age	Target Heart Rate About 60–80% Maximum Beats per Minute	Average Maximum Heart Rate 220 – Age Beats per Minute*
20	120–160	200
25	117–156	195
30	114–152	190

35	111–148	185
40	108–144	180
45	105–140	175

* Source: *Getting in Shape After Your Baby.* Washington, D.C.: American College of Obstetricians and Gynecologists, January 2000.

ACTIVITIES TO PROMOTE AEROBIC ENDURANCE

Swimming, bicycling, brisk walking, jogging, and aerobic dancing are all good activities for new mothers if the heart-rate guidelines are followed. To get the health benefits of these activities, exercise for fifteen to twenty minutes three times a week.

Since most of us exercise unsupervised and at home, it's important to recognize our bodies' trouble signals. The first rule is that if it hurts, don't do it. If you still believe in the no-pain-no-gain theory of exercise, you've been misled. The key to successful exercise is consistency. A workout that causes muscle pain, strain, or fatigue can't hold a sweat band to three days of gentle, satisfying brisk walking.

Warning Signs and Symptoms for New Moms

Stop exercising and call your health care provider if you experience any of the following:

Pain	Faintness
Bleeding	Irregular heartbeats
Dizziness	Back pain
Shortness of breath	Pubic pain
Palpitations	Difficulty walking

WHEN CAN I BEGIN EXERCISE IF I HAD A CESAREAN BIRTH?

This is definitely a question you must ask your doctor. Healing times and medical complications vary from woman to woman. Don't push it. If you feel good and your doctor says you are in good shape and you have the energy, then up to six or more weeks postpartum you may be able to begin an appropriate activity. Walking is a good start.

Remember that in addition to having a baby, you had major surgery. Take care of yourself, but don't think of yourself as an invalid, either. Appropriate exercise and movement can promote healing and recovery.

WHAT IS A GOOD EXERCISE REGIMEN?

Exercise is easy to put off but your muscles are not stagnant; they actually "melt" away if not used. The good news is that it is never too late to start exercising. Aim to exercise every day so if you fail at this daily goal (and most of us do), you will still be active three or four times a week instead of just once. Exercise is not just for weight control. Even more important is what it does for your emotional health. Being active can help fight depression. The next time you are feeling blue, try taking a walk and see if it makes your mood better. A good workout program should include exercise that gets your heart up to its target rate, to provide overall conditioning. Add a gentle strength-training program twice a week. It's also a good idea to do some abdomen-strengthening exercises, because good strong stomach muscles support your back and can help prevent back injuries. I like Miriam Nelson's website, www.strongwomen.com, for step-by-step guidance on a safe strength-training program that suits your level of fitness.

EXERCISES FOR YOUR ABDOMEN

Pelvic Tilt

1. Stand with your feet shoulder-width apart. Bend your knees slightly.
2. Contract the muscles of your abdomen, buttocks, and pelvis. Gently thrust forward, rotating your pubic bone upward. Imagine that you are moving your pubic bone up toward your navel. Hold this position for ten seconds, then release. Repeat ten times.

This can be performed while lying down.

Crunches or the New Safe Sit-Up

The sit-up that we all remember from gym class is no longer recommended as an abdomen toner. The old sit-ups only partially exercised the abdominal muscles while putting lots of strain on the back. Performed correctly, the crunch tightens the tummy without hurting the back.

1. Lie on your back, bend your knees, and keep your feet on the floor.
2. Put your hands at your sides (you can gently hold on to your thighs) or cross them over your chest. (In time you can increase the difficulty of the crunch by crossing your arms over your head and allowing each hand to gently touch the opposite shoulder.)
3. Contract your stomach muscles, press your lower back into the floor, and lift your upper body up to a thirty-five- or forty-five-degree angle.
4. Keep your lower back pressed to the ground without arching and gently return to the floor. Repeat five times. Gently work up to three sets of five.

Many of us perform crunches the wrong way. While "crunching," keep the following in mind:

- To keep your neck properly extended, your chin should not touch your chest. There should always be enough room between your chin and chest to fit a fist or an orange there.
- Don't keep your eyes locked on the ceiling. When you're tightening your abdominal muscles and lifting your head, look at your knees. This will help you stay in the correct position.
- Don't forget to breathe and exhale as you lift.
- If you are placing your hands on your chest and your neck feels tight or strained, place one or both hands under your neck for support.
- Perform crunches in a slow, controlled manner. Fast and jerky is not your goal. This is more like an isometric exercise than an aerobic one.

BACK STRENGTHENING

Many mothers have trouble with their backs while pregnant. Exercise now may help prevent future back troubles. The pelvic tilt described in the abdominal exercises is a good back strengthener. There are also some exercises geared specifically to the back.

Lower-Back Stretch

1. Lie on your back.
2. Take hold of one knee with both hands and pull it toward your chin. Keep the other leg on the floor, straight. Count to ten, then switch legs.

The Side-to-Side

1. Lie on your back with your knees slightly bent.
2. Gently drop your knees to the right while turning your body and both arms to the left.
3. Bring your knees to the upright position and drop to the opposite side.

Cat Stretch

1. Get down on all fours, hands and knees shoulder-width apart.
2. Slowly press your navel toward the floor, allowing your lower back to curve down while you lift your head. Return to neutral.
3. Gently arch your back while you lower your head. Return to neutral.
4. Repeat ten times.

STRETCHING GUIDELINES

Maintaining flexibility is a great way to prevent injury. There are many stretches you can perform while doing household activities or watching TV. One of my favorite books on this subject is *Stretching* by Bob Anderson (Shelter Publications, Inc., 1980).

Here are some guidelines for safe stretching:

- Stop if there's pain.
- Try to stretch three or four times a week.
- Don't bounce when you stretch.
- Hold a stretch in a comfortable position, thirty to sixty seconds.
- Breathe slowly. Exhale as you begin the stretch.

A NEW MOTHER'S EXERCISE ROUTINE

Here's a sample of a safe, healthy exercise plan I used when I was a new mother:

- Monday—Thirty-minute walk (five-minute warm-up, twenty minutes in target-heart-rate zone, five-minute cool-down). Stretch.

- Tuesday—Abdomen and back exercises: crunches, pelvic tilt, cat stretch.
- Wednesday—Thirty-minute ride on exercise bike (five-minute warm-up, twenty minutes in THR zone, five-minute cool-down).
- Thursday—Take the day off.
- Friday—Thirty-minute exercise to a video,* TV show, or the ACOG exercise tape. Most exercise programs have the warm-up and cool-down in the workout.
- Saturday and Sunday—Brisk walk; back and abdomen exercises.

Throughout the day, try pulling in your abdomen muscles and holding them for ten seconds. Do this as often as you remember—perhaps each time you change the baby's diaper.

IS IT SAFE FOR BREASTFEEDING MOTHERS TO EXERCISE?

This is a good question, since a mother who is quite active can use up calories and may also worry about fatigue. The good news is that exercise appears to be compatible with breastfeeding and may even have some desirable effects on lactation.

Cheryl A. Lovelady, Ph.D., R.D., a nutrition researcher, has studied the impact that exercise has on breastfeeding. She and her colleagues recruited sixteen breastfeeding mothers; half were very active, the others were sedentary. Their babies were all between nine and twenty-four weeks old. Each mother was asked to keep a food-and-activity diary. Mothers also collected milk samples for nutrition testing and measured milk volume by using

---

*Most videotapes and TV exercise shows aren't geared for new mothers, so proceed slowly. When bouncing or jumping exercises are part of the routine, walk in place. New mothers may still have more elasticity in their joints and too much bouncing could cause injury, so take it easy.

a sophisticated scale to weigh their babies before and after feedings.

The active mothers participated in aerobic activity (usually swimming, but some jogged or biked) five days a week for forty-five minutes. They expended about 3,200 calories daily and ate 2,700. The sedentary mothers ate about 2,100 calories and expended about 2,400 calories while carrying out their usual activities. The very active mothers experienced no adverse effect on their breastfeeding; in fact, they had higher milk volumes than the sedentary moms. In another study Dr. Lovelady, in collaboration with Kathryn Dewey, Ph.D. and other researchers at the University of California, investigated whether regular exercise had an effect on the amount or quality of breast milk. This time the researchers compared the breast milk of sedentary new mothers and new mothers who exercised forty-five minutes five days per week. They concluded in this study that the mothers who started exercising six to eight weeks postpartum had no adverse reactions while breastfeeding and improved their fitness level.

A study by Megan McCrory that evaluated weight loss in breastfeeding moms by diet alone or diet along with exercise found that losing about two pounds per week by diet plus exercise was safe and may even be better because it maintained lean body mass. These results suggest that it is fine for new breastfeeding mothers to resume vigorous exercise. However, activity and life with a new baby is very personal; only you know what is right while you are breastfeeding and adjusting to your new baby. Keep in mind that the first four to six weeks are when mother and baby bond and become a nursing couple. Both of you need this time to learn to nurse. For some mothers, a time-consuming, vigorous exercise program could compromise this relationship. Use common sense when deciding when to begin your postnatal exercise routine.

If you exercise regularly and vigorously, you must eat enough to meet the demands of exercise and to produce an adequate supply of breast milk. In most cases, if a mother responds to her appetite and hunger pangs, she'll meet her caloric needs. Exercise while breastfeeding has other unique issues. Some mothers find their infants to be fussy and reject nursing even four to six hours after strenuous activity. Sweat is high in salt and chloride, and lactic acid, a by-product of exercise, has a bitter/sour taste. Fussiness after activity might be caused by the effect sweat and lactic acid have on the sensory experience of breastfeeding. Dr. Ruth Lawrence suggests the following guidelines for active moms:

- Shower or wash breasts to remove perspiration before nursing.
- Express a small amount of breast milk manually and discard before feeding.
- If your baby puts on a "pucker face," consider postponing breastfeeding and serve previously pumped milk.

PICK A GOOD SPORTS BRA

When engaging in any kind of vigorous activity, wear a sports bra. Choose one made of cotton; synthetic materials can trap moisture and cause irritation. Buy a bra with wide straps and lots of support.

When I was exercising and nursing I found that a sports bra alone didn't do the trick, so I wore two bras. I wore my nursing bra underneath and put the exercise bra on top. This gave me the extra support I needed.

Ten Thousand Steps

Wear a pedometer and you may find you get more exercise than you thought. Each two thousand steps equals approximately one mile. America on the Move is a national organization dedicated to helping individuals live healthier lives. They have an online site, free as of this writing, in which you can register to track your walking. It is not geared toward new moms, but it is great at providing support. For more information about the ten-thousand-step program, go to www.americaonthemove.org.

WHAT ABOUT INCLUDING MY BABY IN MY EXERCISE ROUTINE?

In an effort to get exercise, a lot of us are bringing our babies along. Exercise can be a wonderful chance to interact with a baby and expose him to some fresh air and new scenery. Exercising with a baby is not without its downside, however. A June 1990 article in *The Physician and Sportsmedicine* cited the following potential risks associated with including your baby in an exercise routine:

- Swimming classes, even conducted under the watchful eye of a parent and instructor, can allow the baby to consume an excessive and potentially dangerous amount of water. Infants may also pick up intestinal parasites such as giardia or viruses that can be transmitted through pool water. Adults are less susceptible to these invaders than babies.
- Jogging with a baby in a stroller can result in a fall or a collision with other runners, animals, bicycles, or even cars.
- Backpack-type carriers used for jogging may jar and shake a young infant's head, causing brain damage. Even a bike ride over very bumpy terrain is risky with a young infant.
- In chilly weather, a baby joining you in outdoor exercise may become too cold and not be able to communicate the problem to you.
- Exercising in the heat or overexposure to the sun has risks as well, such as sunburn and dehydration.
- Hiking in the wilderness could become a nightmare if emergency help is needed for a serious bug bite or injury.

This all sounds very scary, but you need to be aware of any potential risks if you want to include your baby in your activities. You *can* exercise with your baby, but use good judgment.

In response to the article in *The Physician and Sportsmedicine*, Linda Pescatello, an exercising mom in New Britain, Connecticut, wrote a letter to the editor suggesting the following guide-lines for parents who use baby joggers. They sound worthwhile, so I pass them along to you.

1. Avoid using the jogger during environmental extremes, such as hot and humid or cold and blustery weather.
2. Avoid traffic by using the jogger in a park, during a race, or in the early morning hours.
3. Avoid bumpy terrain until the baby is at least one year old. If rough surfaces are unavoidable, deflate the jogger's tires slightly.
4. Use the jogger only when your baby is at least six months old.
5. Use a bicycle helmet to protect your baby's head.
6. Use a canopy and sunblock to protect your baby from the sun.
7. Never push yourself to exhaustion.

RELAXATION

There's more to good health than just exercising and eating well. Allowing time for relaxation can go a long way toward promoting well-being. For me, a new baby added quite a bit of stress to my life. I felt as though I was always rushing to do something while I managed our home and cared for our family. Relaxation techniques helped me cope with this stress.

Relaxation therapy isn't really exercise, but it's important for new mothers. As a breastfeeding mom, you can try some relaxation techniques while you feed your baby. You may both fall asleep, but that's okay. (If you do tend to fall asleep, you may want to doze off after you've switched breasts. Otherwise you may be lopsided from feeding your baby on just one side.) Two relaxation techniques—imagery and deep breathing—can give new moms much-needed relief from stress.

Imagery

While you're nursing, make yourself comfortable. Close your eyes and imagine a beautiful scene. Look at every detail. If you're in a garden, look at every flower. Visualize the colors. Imagine how it would feel to walk on soft, cool grass. Imagine how the air would smell. Can you hear birds? Is the sky blue? Are clouds gliding by? Are you sitting or lying down?

Deep Breathing

Make yourself comfortable sitting or lying down, in a position you won't have to move out of too soon. Then take a deep breath, slowly exhale, and breathe in again gently. With each breath you exhale, think of a number (you can count backward or repeat the same number over and over). Continue breathing. Each time you exhale, think of a number and allow the number to push away all other thoughts that try to creep in. Do this for as long as you can. It may be only five minutes. The next day, try it again and see if you can go just a bit longer. If not, that's okay, too. Just that little bit of time you allow your mind to relax can affect your whole body and your well-being.

I FEEL LIKE A FAILURE

For lots of us, exercise is an all-or-nothing commitment. We set goals for exercising three to four times a week, we meet these goals for a week or two, and then we stop. Our usual response is that we failed. We feel guilty, and that's the end of the exercise program—until we get concerned again about our weight or health and make new commitments, carry them out for a week or two, and let them, too, fall by the wayside.

Here's my advice: assume that your exercise routine will always be in transition and that there will be weeks when you meet all your goals and weeks when you won't. Just keep doing it. You aren't a failure because you didn't exercise.

SPEAK POSITIVELY

You aren't alone if the desire to exercise doesn't come naturally. Over my career as a dietitian, I have talked to literally thousands of people about exercising more. It is a rare client who approaches exercise with enthusiasm. Most of the time I hear comments like, "I know I should, but I just can't find the time." Instead of thinking of exercise as an additional burden, try to see it as a privilege. Start speaking positively about it and tell friends and family: "Boy, I love to get out and take my walks" or "It feels so good to get out and move" or "Gee, since I started to exercise more I really do feel better."

Try speaking and thinking positively about exercising, and you may even find it's more of a pleasure than a burden.

8

NO, NO, NOT NOW—
KEEPING BREAST MILK
SAFE FOR YOUR BABY

As new parents we pay attention to every little burp, coo, and cry our babies make. It's likely that while you're breastfeeding, you'll be more concerned with what you eat than at any other time in your life. Breastfeeding moms almost always try to analyze how meals affect their babies. If the baby is up at night, the mom blames the spicy spaghetti sauce at dinner or the chocolate bar she snacked on after lunch.

When our babies are fussy or crying, we try to determine what we ate that we shouldn't have so that we can remove the offending substance from our diets. The truth is that little babies cry and they cry and then they cry some more. Most of the time our babies cry in reaction to something completely unrelated to what we have eaten. But sometimes, what we eat does affect how our babies feel.

Concern about eating well while breastfeeding is indeed a good thing, but don't be too hard on yourself. Some mothers won't go near a cup of coffee, or they completely restrict the salt and spices in their food. This chapter will explore the facts behind the food myths that have surrounded the diets of breastfeeding mothers for generations. In most cases, moderation is the key to a happy mother and a happy baby. But there are some things moms do need to be cautious about, including caffeine, alcohol, drugs, and pesticides.

CAN I EAT IT?

It's not uncommon to gather with a group of nursing mothers for lunch and hear questions about the menu like "What's in it?" "Does it have garlic?" "Are there onions in this?"

It's true that what we eat affects our health and breast milk, but there is no scientific evidence that foods that cause gas in you create gas in your baby. Even if you eat a big bowl of beans and feel discomfort yourself, the gas in your intestinal tract does not go into your bloodstream and it does not get into your breast milk. Foods that give you gas aren't going to do the same to your baby.

Foods like oranges, grapefruit, or tomatoes are often thought of as too acidic for a baby. Again, there's no evidence to support this. Once you eat an acidic food, it mixes with your digestive juices and reaches the pH (acid level) that's right for your body. An acidic food cannot change the pH of your blood or your breast milk.

A complex system of checks and balances keeps your body in harmony even when you eat large servings of certain foods. Yes, you may find that some foods eaten by you do affect the baby. If so, eliminate the food and try it again a week or so later. If it bothers the baby again, stay away from it. If it doesn't bother the baby again, the connection the first time around may have been just a coincidence.

Researchers at the University of Minnesota mailed questionnaires to 272 breastfeeding mothers to ask if their diet affected their baby's colic symptoms. The moms responded that cruciferous vegetables (cabbage, Brussels sprouts, cauliflower, and broccoli), cow's milk, onions, and chocolate were associated with colic symptoms. The researchers concluded that it may be reasonable to exclude these foods in exclusively breastfeeding women whose babies have colic symptoms.

Eliminating the limited list of vegetables above or chocolate won't be a problem, but restricting cow's milk if it is a mother's primary source of calcium requires that an alternate calcium source be added. There is no harm in eliminating or temporarily avoiding a few foods while you breastfeed. The danger comes only if you eliminate whole food groups such as dairy, citrus fruits, or wheat products.

One fascinating report might actually encourage mothers to try more flavorful foods. In 1991 researcher Dr. Julie Mennella at the Monell Chemical Senses Center in Philadelphia asked eight breastfeeding mothers to eat garlic extract capsules before nursing their babies. The capsules significantly changed the odor of the mothers' milk. Instead of the garlic being a deterrent, the babies actually nursed longer and consumed more milk than they did when their mothers ate a relatively bland diet. This research suggests that flavorful foods should not be eliminated from the breastfeeding mother's menu. In fact, the researchers speculate that early exposure to a variety of flavors in breast milk may increase a baby's willingness to try a greater variety of foods as a child.

Almost all the reports of foods eaten by a mother affecting her baby are anecdotal stories; I couldn't find any hard research evidence. In *Breastfeeding: A Guide for the Medical Profession*, Dr. Ruth Lawrence reports that the natural oils in some foods such as garlic and some spices have flavors and odors that might be capable of passing into breast milk and upsetting a baby. Garlic, onions, cabbage, turnips, broccoli, dried beans, rhubarb, apricots, and prunes are all mentioned by Dr. Lawrence as potential causes of colic, as is a heavy diet of fresh fruits and melons. Red pepper has been identified as a cause of dermatitis because of the naturally occurring capsaicin it contains. These foods are commonly cited by mothers as being troublesome and since I trust the collective wisdom of experienced moms, I suspect there is probably some validity to the list. Mothers know their bodies best. Just don't be a slave to what works for other women.

Dr. Lawrence described another interesting effect food can

have on breast milk. Breast milk is usually a bluish white to creamy white color. One mother's breast milk turned pink-orange from the dyes used in the orange soda she routinely drank; fresh beets may do the same. Other mothers have reported green milk from drinking Gatorade, taking some medications, or eating kelp, other seaweeds, and certain vitamins from the health food store. Dr. Lawrence has written about two reports of black milk caused by a medication also capable of causing black pigmentation of the skin. To get rid of an unusual color, the mother's diet must be scrutinized and the coloring agent avoided. No health risks to the baby from colored milk are known, but certainly it's best to avoid these chemicals.

CAN I DRINK COFFEE?

When I first started to nurse Sarah, one of the first changes I made in my diet was to eliminate regular coffee. The caffeine in coffee is a stimulant, showing up in breast milk within thirty minutes, and I didn't want Sarah to be any more wakeful, particularly at night, than she already was. Much later, when I started to research some of the particulars about what mothers should and should not eat, I found that caffeine, in small amounts, wasn't that bad. But it can pose a problem if consumed in large amounts.

One cup of regular coffee won't harm your baby, but in the United States coffee drinkers average three cups per day. Your body quickly absorbs the 150 milligrams of caffeine in a cup of coffee, but only about 1 to 5 milligrams of that caffeine will end up in a full liter of your breast milk. This is a very small amount, but there is a catch. In the adult body, caffeine stays in the bloodstream for only three to five hours before it's excreted. It can remain in your baby's blood for eighty hours—up to ninety-seven hours for preterm infants. This means that infants can accumulate caffeine. One cup of coffee a day shouldn't cause trouble, but a mother drinking more than three cups a day may start to have an irritable, wakeful baby.

Caffeine is found not only in coffee (see table 8). Tea and dark colas can be significant caffeine sources if you drink them frequently.

Table 8. Caffeine Content of Selected Beverages

Coffee
Brewed drip, 6 ounces	103 mg
Instant, 6 ounces	57 mg
Decaffeinated	2 mg

Tea
Black, 5 ounces	36 mg
Iced, 8 ounces, from instant powder	31 mg

Sodas
Coca Cola classic, 8 ounces	35 mg
Mellow Yellow, 8 ounces	35 mg
Mountain Dew, 8 ounces	55 mg
Pepsi, 8 ounces	37 mg
Cocoa mix, 5 ounces	4 mg
Chocolate milk, 8 ounces	8 mg
Dark chocolate, 1 ounce	17 mg
Milk chocolate, 1 ounce	7 mg

Switching to decaffeinated coffee can certainly reduce your caffeine intake, but it doesn't seem to be just the caffeine in coffee that's the problem. A study of breastfeeding mothers drinking more than three cups of coffee per day while they were pregnant and breastfeeding found that the concentrations of iron in the mothers' breast milk was low and their babies' own iron status was compromised. Coffee's effect on iron doesn't seem to be linked to caffeine but to some other chemical component.

Because of coffee's adverse effects on breastfeeding babies, it's best if you drink only one to two cups a day and keep your total daily caffeine intake below 300 milligrams.

CHOCOLATE—THE FOOD WE HATE OURSELVES FOR LOVING

Chocolate is surrounded by folklore. Mothers who eat chocolate while breastfeeding fear they'll cause their babies diarrhea, irritability, even eczema. Though there are many anecdotal reports about how chocolate is thought to affect babies, hard evidence is scarce.

One 1977 study seems to take chocolate off the breastfeeding mothers' "no" list. Beth Resman, Pharm.D., a researcher at the State University of New York at Buffalo, asked six breastfeeding mothers to eat a single four-ounce serving of Hershey's milk chocolate. She found that none of the infants in her study experienced any adverse effect when their mothers ate this moderate portion of chocolate. If you love chocolate, go ahead and eat a small amount—I don't want you to feel deprived, and your baby probably won't mind. But if you are convinced that chocolate bothers your baby, then by all means stay away from it.

Why Do We Love Chocolate?

Many women complain of being chocoholics, particularly around their periods. There may be some scientific reason for this. It seems that our need for calories increases during our menstrual cycle, and bingeing on chocolate, a concentrated source of calories, may be a way to meet that need.

Chocolate may also act like a mood-altering drug. It's rich in substances that raise our spirits and make us feel better. I know chocolate makes me feel better. I love the way it tastes and smells. Chocolate is now being credited with health benefits such as lowering blood pressure and even helping to improve insulin sensitivity. But it is rich in calories, over 100 calories per ounce. To balance desire with moderation I treat myself on special occasions to really good chocolate or I make homemade chocolate sauce. You can try the fat-free chocolate sauce I use as my occasional treat—the recipe is on page 199.

If heartburn is a problem for you, chocolate might be a food to avoid. Chocolate and other foods such as alcohol, coffee, spearmint, peppermint, and those with high fat are thought to increase heartburn symptoms.

IS IT SAFE TO TAKE MEDICATIONS WHILE BREASTFEEDING?

Many drugs pass into breast milk; some could cause your child discomfort or even harm. Always check with your physician before taking any prescription medication. Have a frank discussion with your doctor and make sure he knows you're breastfeeding. Your doctor may advise you to take the medication at a particular time, like after your baby has nursed. This way the medication may no longer be as active in your bloodstream and breast milk by the next feeding.

Herbs and Herbal Treatment

Many of today's medications drew their roots from herbal remedies. Just as you would not take a medication without ensuring it had no effect on breast milk, be as thoughtful regarding the use of herbs. *Natural* is not synonymous with *safe* and there are no FDA controls, so be sure to check with your child's pediatrician before using them while breastfeeding. Good websites for more information include Consumer Laboratories (www.consumerlab. com) and National Center for Complementary and Alternative Medicine (http://nccam.nih.gov).

IS IT SAFE TO DRINK ALCOHOL WHILE BREASTFEEDING?

Your own common sense will have already told you that heavy drinking is absolutely unacceptable while breastfeeding.

The alcohol you drink passes from your stomach to your bloodstream. If you drink only a small amount, your liver can quickly remove the alcohol from your blood. But if you drink a lot, your liver can't keep up, and your blood levels will get even higher with each sip. The alcohol in your blood can pass into your breast milk. If there's a lot of alcohol in your blood, then not only do you get drunk—so does your baby.

Besides causing drunkenness, excess alcohol can interfere with oxytocin, the chemical that controls milk ejection. Excess alcohol consumption can thus slow the delivery of milk to your baby.

Okay, so you know that getting drunk isn't advised, but what about a glass of wine with supper? It has long been thought that the occasional glass of wine or cold beer can help a mother relax and thus actually assist in the letdown reflex and breastfeeding itself. Studies have shown that within thirty minutes of drinking a small amount of alcohol, especially beer, a mother's levels of prolactin, the hormone that stimulates milk production, increase significantly.

The 1991 Subcommittee on Nutrition During Lactation suggests that mothers who want to drink while breastfeeding consume not more than 2 to 2.5 ounces of liquor, 8 ounces of wine, or two cans of beer in any one day. These guidelines are designed to protect your baby from becoming intoxicated, but you must remember that a couple of beers each night is going to add a few hundred extra calories (see table 9) and the alcohol is likely to have you quite groggy at that two o'clock feeding. Current public health guidelines recommend moderate drinking for all of us, breastfeeding or not. Moderate alcohol intake is defined as one drink per day and a drink is defined as a 12-ounce beer, 5 ounces of wine, or 1.5 ounces of liquor.

Table 9. Calorie Content of Various Alcoholic Beverages

Regular beer, 12 ounces	151 calories
Light beer, 12 ounces	100 calories*

| 80-proof liquor, 1.5 ounces | 97 calories |
| White wine, 7 ounces | 174 calories |

*This is an estimate. Individual products may vary in caloric content.

When I first began to investigate what mothers should eat and drink while breastfeeding, I was told by one prominent doctor that there was absolutely no evidence that one alcoholic drink consumed by a nursing mother would harm a healthy baby. That was in 1987. Since then, a cloud of suspicion has been cast over the safety of that one drink.

Dr. Ruth Little of the University of Michigan studied four hundred infants to investigate the effects a mother's moderate alcohol intake had on her year-old infant. Dr. Little found that tests designed to measure mental function did not uncover any connection between what the mother drank and how her breastfed baby fared on the test. However, the children whose mothers had at least one drink daily did score lower on motor-development tests than infants who were not exposed to as much alcohol.

The study didn't consider the actual amount of alcohol in the breast milk, socioeconomic variables, or the way the mothers interacted with their children, but it did seem to link moderate maternal alcohol consumption with impaired motor development in children.

In a 2001 study in *Alcoholism: Clinical and Experimental Research*, Julie Mennella, Ph.D., asked twelve nursing mothers to drink orange juice mixed with a small amount of alcohol. The researchers compared how the babies nursed after the alcoholic drink to how they nursed after their mothers drank a glass of plain orange juice. The babies consumed significantly less milk after their mothers drank the orange juice with alcohol. The researchers suspect that alcohol may have an undesirable effect on the flavor of breast milk, diminish the baby's ability or desire to feed, or even decrease milk production.

Sensory tests conducted on the mothers' milk showed that a

change in odor peaked thirty to sixty minutes after they drank the alcohol. This suggests that mothers who know they will be drinking may want to feed their babies before having that drink. Alcohol, whether it is wine, beer, or liquor, must be consumed cautiously by breastfeeding mothers. It provides calories and, if consumed in excess, could harm you and upset your baby. When you do drink, you probably want to avoid breastfeeding for two hours. The alcohol level of breast milk matches your own blood-alcohol level. Only time clears the alcohol from your body; pumping and discarding breast milk will not do it. So if you choose to drink, do so in moderation and after you have nursed.

ILLEGAL DRUGS

The prudent thing to do while breastfeeding is to avoid all drugs, including marijuana and cocaine. The active ingredient in marijuana is tetrahydrocannabinol; once absorbed, this chemical is stored in body fat. Since body fat is used to fuel breast-milk production, a mother who is a heavy marijuana user may have marijuana in her milk. A child ingesting marijuana from breast milk may appear sleepier and become less interested in nursing. Animal studies show that newborn animals drinking mother's milk contaminated with marijuana had alterations in their brain cells. Since your marijuana smoking can have a negative impact on your baby, please don't smoke during the months you breastfeed. Not only can the chemicals harm your baby directly; if you smoke, you won't be fully alert to your baby's needs, either.

If a mother uses cocaine or heroin, it can show up in her milk. It is known that during pregnancy both drugs can have serious negative consequences for the developing baby, such as low birth weight. Common sense should be your guide. Mothers who can't stop using these substances should stop nursing.

Marijuana, alcohol, heroin, and cocaine do more than affect

your body. They affect your mind and your judgment. A baby needs your unclouded attention, and a new mother just can't be at her best if any of these drugs are in the way.

WILL CIGARETTE SMOKE HURT MY BABY?

Cigarette smoking is actively discouraged because of its effect on you and your baby. If you quit smoking while pregnant, please don't take it up again. Once your baby is delivered, it might not seem so important not to smoke, but it still is.

First of all, smoking hurts you. Heavy smokers have more lung and heart disease. The nicotine from cigarettes may also pass into your breast milk and upset your baby. A mother who smokes twenty cigarettes a day can have a high level of fat-soluble nicotine in her breast milk, which could cause nausea and vomiting in her baby. Cigarette smoking can also reduce milk volume because it inhibits prolactin and oxytocin production. Babies with mothers who smoke tend to be weaned sooner and have a greater incidence of colic.

Finally, there is the real problem of secondhand smoke. Even formula-fed babies exposed to secondhand smoke have measurable levels of nicotine in their urine, meaning they are inhaling the cigarette smoke along with the smoker. A child who breathes in a smoke-filled environment may have respiratory problems.

Infrequent smoking is probably okay, but mothers who smoke ten to twenty cigarettes or more each day should definitely quit or try to cut down. At the very least, don't smoke around your baby. Don't let visitors smoke around your baby, either.

A child in a smoking household is more likely to come across matches or lighters that look like toys and are capable of causing serious burns. Parents who smoke can accidentally burn their child with falling ashes. A child may see a lit cigarette and reach for it out of curiosity, with disastrous results. If Mom and Dad smoke, then their child may start the same unhealthy habit when he reaches adolescence.

THE HIDDEN MENACE

As a mother, the dangers that worry me the most are the ones I can't see. Pesticides alarm us because most of us don't understand how they work. And, worst of all, we can't control them. Scientists try to reassure us that the foods we eat are safe, even if they contain pesticides. As a breastfeeding mother, you may feel that your baby is safe from environmental contaminants because he has not yet started on food. The sad truth is that almost all mothers carry contaminants such as polychlorinated biphenyls (PCBs) and dioxin in their bodies. Our babies may even have been exposed to the chemicals as we carried them in our wombs. This exposure probably continues as we breastfeed.

Dioxin is a by-product of chemical manufacturing and incineration, and it has been accumulating in dirt, in riverbeds, and on plants since the 1940s. It accumulates particularly well in fat. When we eat the fish that feed in the rivers or the animals that eat the dioxin-tainted plant foods or the grains grown in soil with dioxin in it, then we ingest the dioxin, too. That dioxin can pass into our breast milk.

The debate continues as to the risk to babies drinking breast milk contaminated with dioxin. One article cited the risks from drinking dioxin-tainted breast milk as minuscule when compared to the risk associated with riding in a car. Commercial formula is virtually dioxin free, but it doesn't offer the health-promoting benefits of breastfeeding and is not recommended as an alternative. In fact, breastfeeding may give babies a developmental edge if methylmercury, another potentially dangerous environmental toxin, is present.

Since dioxin accumulates in fat and other tissues, the best a mother can do is to control her own animal-fat intake and lose weight slowly. Fruits and vegetables contain almost no dioxins. Since milk is in part synthesized from the mother's own stored fat supplies, it is thought that rapid weight loss may increase the concentration of the chemical in her milk. Dr. Cheryl Lovelady conducted a study to find out if weight loss at four to twenty weeks postpartum increased the concentration of contaminants. She found that moderate weight loss in women who had low exposure to contaminants did not increase contaminant concentration in breast milk. Prudent weight loss of no more than four and a half pounds a month is probably still the best path.

In a study published in the *American Journal of Public Health,* Dr. Walter Rogan found that the presence of some chemicals in breast milk may interfere with the length of time a mother breastfeeds. Dr. Rogan began a project in 1978 that measured the content of PCBs and dichlorodiphenyl dichloroethene (DDE, a metabolite of the infamous DDT pesticide) being consumed by 858 children who were breastfed by their mothers. Dr. Rogan found that women with higher concentrations of DDE, and perhaps PCBs, breastfed for a shorter length of time. DDE may have an estrogen-like effect that suppresses lactation. In a *Journal of Pediatrics* 2003 study examining the effect that prenatal PCB exposure had on children at age eleven, adverse effects were found in children who had not been breastfed. It is not clear why breastfeeding defends against pesticides; nutrients or better education of the mothers may be factors. Given that we all live in a polluted world, it is nice to know that breastfeeding, for whatever reason, may offer one more layer of protection.

To reduce your risk of undesirable chemical and pesticide ingestion and to minimize your baby's exposure to these substances, you can:

- Eat a variety of foods so that you limit your exposure from any one food.
- Try to buy foods in season, which can mean they have fewer chemicals on them.
- Buy low-fat dairy products.

- Trim all meats.
- Don't eat poultry skin.
- Bake or broil instead of frying.
- Eat lots of fruits and vegetables.
- Buy local produce or at least produce grown in the United States.
- Wash your produce. Submerge in water and scrub with a vegetable brush.
- Peel waxed foods like cucumbers, peppers, and apples.
- If using orange or lemon peel or zest in a recipe, buy organic fruit.
- Discard the outer leaves of cabbage.
- If your diet is already rich in fiber, peel carrots, peaches, and pears.
- Buy organic.

Ask your supermarket to label the origins of the foods it sells. If they're not labeled, ask the produce manager where the food comes from. He'll know if the fruits and vegetables are from Naples, Florida, or Naples, Italy. Food grown within the United States must comply with U.S. guidelines for pesticide use, and these products are often better regulated than produce from foreign countries.

Fish: Safe or Not

The health benefits of fish cannot be ignored. Fish contains a rich source of essential fatty acids that are essential to brain and nerve development and the prevention of heart disease. However, almost all fish contain traces of methylmercury, and some farm-raised fish may carry high levels of PCBs. Methylmercury can potentially damage the nervous system and brain development. PCBs are thought to be carcinogens. Particularly vulnerable individuals include pregnant women and young children. The University of Albany released a 2004 study on contaminants in "Farmed vs. Wild Salmon" and recommended consuming farmed salmon in only limited amounts: "Even one or two meals of farmed salmon per month may exceed acceptable contaminant levels." Their full report can be accessed at www.albany.edu/ihe/salmonstudy/consumers.html.

You might think eliminating fish would be an acceptable solution, but it isn't. Eliminating all fish means you and your baby will be missing out on the health benefits contained in marine oils. The CSPI wrote in 2004, "Experts estimate that the heart-healthy omega-3 fats in wild or farmed salmon can save at least 300 lives for every one death from cancer caused by the contamination in salmon." Both the public and the press have responded with great alarm to the reports about contamination in farmed salmon. I am hopeful that the farmed salmon industry will respond with self-regulation and will offer reassurance in the near future to young families about the use of their products. Until then, women of childbearing age and young children need to be particularly careful about their fish intake. Avoid those on the Environmental Protection Agency (EPA) list but do rotate between fish on the "Lower Levels of Mercury" list and buy canned tuna labeled "chunk light" instead of "white (albacore)." Choose fresh, frozen, or canned wild salmon instead of farmed salmon. According to CSPI, wild salmon is best, followed by farmed Atlantic salmon from Chile or Washington state, then other farmed salmon from the United States, Canada, and Norway. Try the Salmon Croquettes on page 186 using canned salmon labeled "wild."

The EPA suggests women who may become pregnant, pregnant women, nursing mothers, and young children should avoid certain fish and shellfish and follow these recommendations:

1. Do not eat shark, swordfish, king mackerel, or tilefish because they contain high levels of mercury.
2. Eat up to twelve ounces (two average meals; children can eat smaller amounts) a week of a variety of fish and shellfish that are lower in mercury. These include catfish, clams, cod, blue king crab, snow crab, haddock, herring, lobster, pollock, scallops, shrimp, and canned light tuna.

The full report along with a complete list of high- and low-mercury–containing fish can be accessed at www.cfsan.fda.gov/~dms/admehg3.html.

Alcohol, drugs, and too much caffeine could all be passed on to your baby. While breastfeeding, you must be cautious but not fanatical. There are still plenty of good foods and nonalcoholic drinks to be enjoyed so you won't feel deprived. Eat a wide variety of food and let common sense guide you when making decisions about what you will put in your mouth.

9

SPECIAL PROBLEMS—
SPECIFIC ANSWERS

Cesarean birth, returning to work, diabetes, vegetarian menus, allergies, anemias, hemorrhoids, and premature births are just a few of the issues that breastfeeding mothers may have to deal with. Eating properly can help a mother cope successfully with these special situations.

ALLERGIES

Each year fifty million Americans are affected by allergies, accounting for more than sixteen million doctor's visits. Approximately 8 percent of children below age six will experience a food allergy. If you have a family history of allergies, your decision to breastfeed is a good one. Breastfeeding alone doesn't guarantee that your child won't get an allergy, but it does appear to reduce the risk and postpone onset. Breast milk may protect babies against allergies by boosting their immune systems, and mothers may be able to pass on some of their own allergy-fighting substances to their babies in their milk. A baby is most likely to develop a food allergy when she is between four and nine months old. By breastfeeding and delaying the introduction of solid foods until a child is four to six months old, you will reduce her chance of developing a food allergy. Protein is the substance in food that triggers an allergic reaction. For this reason, protein-rich foods are usually delayed until a baby is eight or nine months old. Breast milk supplies plenty of protein for young infants and babies.

Foods Most Likely to Cause Allergies

Eggs
Milk and other dairy products
Peanuts
Soybeans
Wheat
Fish

Since the late 1970s, researchers have been investigating whether the foods a mother eats can help prevent allergies in her child. Several studies are now available that demonstrate that what a breastfeeding mother eats can affect her child's risk for allergies. Proteins are common allergy offenders. Mothers with a strong family history of allergies may want to limit the amount of common allergens she eats, such as wheat and eggs. The protein a mother eats may cross over into the milk she produces and precipitate an allergic reaction in her baby.

In a study by Ranjit Chandra, M.D., published in *Clinical Allergy,* 109 mothers completed a research project that followed them through pregnancy and lactation. All the mothers had an older child with an allergy or eczema. Half were assigned a diet that restricted their intake of potentially problematic foods such as dairy products, eggs, fish, beef, and peanuts. The other half were given no food restrictions.

Dr. Chandra confirmed that mothers avoiding the common allergenic foods during pregnancy and lactation had children with a lower incidence of allergies and less severe cases of allergic disease. Children of the women on the restricted diet had fewer incidences of eczema; when it did occur, the eczema was milder than that of the children whose mothers did not restrict their diets. Even the babies born to mothers who followed the restricted diet while pregnant but chose formula over breast milk had less severe cases of eczema.

Before mothers with family histories of allergies start restricting every potentially problematic food, we have to look beyond the study group and statistics to see how this translates to individuals. Of the fifty-five mothers on the avoidance diet, seventeen had babies who developed eczema; of the fifty-four mothers on the regular diet, twenty-four had babies who developed eczema. Statistically, there is a measurable difference in these two groups, but the restricted diet didn't eliminate the risk of allergy. Even though this study and others like it show that a percentage of mothers and babies may be helped by a restricted diet, that diet will not benefit all mothers and their babies.

Imagine, too, how difficult it would be to avoid eggs, dairy products, and beef. Also think of the changes in the nutritional quality of your diet if you eliminated these protein-rich foods. Of course, if it would protect your baby against a lifelong battle with allergies, I know you're thinking it might be worth it.

The Subcommittee on Nutrition During Lactation advises mothers not to eliminate whole food groups to prevent allergies unless there is evidence that the mother is "sensitive or intolerant to the food or that the breastfed infant reacts to the food ingested by the mother."

A mother who suspects her breastfed baby is allergic to a particular food she's eating may want to try an elimination diet under the supervision of her doctor. In this case the offending food is taken out of the mother's diet to see if the baby's symptoms disappear. Then the food is reintroduced under careful supervision to determine whether the symptoms reappear. If they do, the culprit has been exposed. If the food must be eliminated for weeks or months, then the mother will have to do some special dietary planning. For example, if she must eliminate eggs, she can make up for the lost protein by substituting meat, cheese, or fish. A diet void of all the potentially problematic foods is not recommended on a preventative basis for mothers because it is not found to help all babies and it could compromise the nutritional status of the mothers.

CAN I CONTROL COLIC BY WHAT I EAT?

Colic is one of the most frustrating problems parents have with infants. It affects about 20 percent of all babies. For no reason that can be determined, a happy, smiling baby starts to cry. His legs pull up, his fists clench, his face turns red, and he screams in pain for an hour or more. As quickly as it starts, it can stop. Holding the baby upright or laying him, tummy side down, on a warm water bottle may help. Often, nothing works to calm him except time. These crying bouts seem to occur most frequently in the late afternoon or early evening, usually when a baby is between six weeks and three months old.

No one knows for sure, but these crying jags may be caused by an immaturity in a baby's newly working digestive tract that can cause spasm or cramps. There is a lot of talk about how a mother's diet can affect colic symptoms, but not a lot of research. Dr. Irene Jakobsson from the University of Lund in Sweden has published two studies on this problem.

In her first study published in 1978 in The Lancet, Dr. Jakobsson asked eighteen mothers with colicky babies to eat a milk-free diet. Almost immediately the colic disappeared in thirteen of the babies; symptoms reappeared in twelve of the babies when their mothers started drinking milk again. In a later study published in the journal Pediatrics, Dr. Jakobsson studied sixty-six mothers and their colicky babies. Again she found that when mothers were put on a milk-free diet, the colic disappeared in thirty-five of the breastfed infants, reappearing in twenty-three of those infants when their mothers started drinking milk again.

Dr. Jakobsson has concluded that in one-third of breastfed infants, colic is related to cow's milk consumption by the mother and that when colic is a problem, mothers should try a milk-free diet. It is believed that part of the cow's milk protein that the mother drinks passes into her breast milk. Some infants may have trouble digesting this form of protein, and colic is the result.

Another study sheds even more light on cow's milk and colic. Dr. Patrick Clyne and Dr. Anthony Kulczycki reported in the journal *Pediatrics* on their study of twenty-nine mothers of colicky babies and thirty mothers with babies the same age who did not have colic. The mothers who had colicky babies had much higher levels of cow antibodies in their breast milk than the other mothers. These antibodies are proteins that occur in small amounts in cow's milk. Until this study, only the larger proteins in cow's milk had been examined as a cause of colic. It appears that the more milk a mother drinks, the more cow's milk antibodies she will ingest and pass on to her baby through her own milk. Cow's milk antibodies can also be found in formula made from cow's milk. This helps to explain why colic occurs equally in bottle-fed babies and breastfed babies.

Milk may not be the only culprit. When questionnaires about colic and diet were mailed to breastfeeding mothers of four-month-old infants, a significant number of the mothers associated their intake of cruciferous vegetables, onions, and chocolate as well as cow's milk with colic symptoms in their infants. These mothers did not associate eating beans, legumes, spicy foods, or caffeine with the same degree of colic symptoms.

Why all babies don't get colic and why only some are helped when their mother stops drinking cow's milk is unknown. Colic probably has other causes, including psychological ones. So don't just worry about what you're eating; give some good old-fashioned hugs and cuddles, too. If it seems like your baby is anxious to nurse, then refuses to feed when put to the breast, it may be that she smells the milk and acts as if she wants to nurse when she really does not. Try having someone else (a nonnursing mother) hold her to see if that calms her down. It never hurts to reassure and comfort a child, but remember: babies cry a lot—

about two to two and a half hours every day. And whatever you do, or don't do, your baby will probably outgrow colic symptoms by the time he's three months old.

SHOULD I STOP DRINKING MILK?

There just isn't enough evidence to make an across-the-board recommendation that mothers should reduce their cow's milk consumption to avoid or eliminate colic. If colic is a problem, a temporary elimination of milk for one week can be tried (one day will not do it). If Dr. Jakobsson is right that 30 percent of colicky breastfed babies can get relief if their mothers eliminate milk, then it's worth a try. The colic should correct itself by the time your baby is three months old, at which time you can start eating milk products again.

The problem with eliminating milk is that it puts you at even greater risk of not meeting your calcium needs. After all, it's difficult for mothers to meet the calcium recommendation even if they are milk drinkers. Fortunately, calcium is added to a lot of foods, such as juice and even bread products.

IF I CAN'T DRINK MILK, WHAT SHOULD I DO?

Some mothers can't drink milk. They may have a milk allergy or an inability to digest the milk sugar called lactose. If lactose intolerance is your problem, you can find help by using Lactaid, an over-the-counter product that contains an enzyme that predigests lactose so that you don't have to. Lactaid milk and cheeses, which are as rich in calcium and protein as regular cow's milk products, are also available (look in the Resources section for suggestions on where to find Lactaid products). Lactaid milk and cheeses still contain cow's milk proteins, so they are not products for people with milk allergies.

Mothers who are allergic to milk or who are on a self-imposed milk-free diet must do some careful planning. A milk-free diet means no yogurt, cheese, ice cream, buttermilk, or cottage cheese, which eliminates some of your very best calcium sources. These mothers will need to eat lots of nondairy calcium-rich foods (see table 10) or take an appropriate supplement.

Table 10. Calcium-Rich Nondairy Foods

The following foods, in the portions listed, provide 300 milligrams of calcium, as much as is contained in 1 cup of milk. The DRI for lactating women is 1,000 milligrams of calcium a day and 1,300 milligrams for women under age eighteen.

Food	Portion providing 300 mg calcium
Sardines with bones	3 ounces
Spinach	1¾ cups cooked
Oysters	6–9 medium
Turnip greens	1¼ cups cooked
Broccoli	2¼ cups cooked
Salmon, canned, with bones	1 cup
Beet greens	2 cups cooked
Orange juice with calcium	8 ounces
Dandelion greens	2 cups cooked
Soybeans	2 cups cooked
Tofu or calcium-fortified soy milk	8 ounces
Collards	¾ cup cooked
Almonds	1 cup chopped

Milk doesn't just provide calcium. It is also a good source of protein, vitamin D, and some of the B vitamins. Be cautious if you consider eliminating it from your diet.

SHOULD I TAKE CALCIUM SUPPLEMENTS?

Calcium supplements fall woefully short on nutrition when compared to milk. They contain only calcium and none of the other nutrients found in milk. Calcium in pills is also not as well absorbed as dietary calcium. But if calcium pills are needed, there are a few things you should know.

Calcium pills are available as calcium carbonate or calcium citrate. Calcium citrate is recommended by the National Institutes of Health as the most efficient way to get calcium because it is well absorbed but many women choose calcium carbonate, found in the antacid Tums, because it is less expensive. This is important because if supplements are your primary source of calcium, you will need to take enough to meet your goal of 1,000 to 1,300 milligrams every day. Regular multivitamin-mineral preparations don't contain this large amount. Multivitamin-mineral supplements are not a recommended way to get the calcium you need because you would probably need to take quite a few of the pills, and then your intake of other nutrients like zinc and vitamins A, D, and B_6 might be excessive.

Though Tums is marketed as a medicine, it is a safe and reliable way to supplement your diet with calcium. Read the label to determine dosage and consider dividing into two doses to reduce the risk of constipation that some women report.

The dosage you need will depend on how many foods with calcium you eat. If you don't eat dairy but eat lots of calcium-rich green leafy vegetables or tofu, you may not need to take a full 1,000 to 1,300 milligrams of calcium pills a day. If kidney stones have plagued you, talk over the use of calcium pills with your doctor. Any mother taking calcium supplements should drink plenty of fluids. This keeps your urine diluted and reduces your risk for kidney stones. You may be able to enhance the absorption of the calcium in your pills by spreading them out through the day instead of taking one large dose. Calcium may interfere with iron absorption, an issue if you are being treated for iron-deficiency anemia. Keep your doctor informed of your supplement use.

Calcium-fortified orange juice, bread, cereals, and even soft drinks are now available in most supermarkets. Any food with 30 percent calcium listed on the label is an excellent calcium source. The Subcommittee on Nutrition During Lactation recommends that mothers who cannot eat milk, cheese, or other dairy products, and cannot eat enough of alternative calcium nondairy foods, should take a supplement of 600 milligrams of elemental calcium per day with meals. At this dosage, calcium is safe. Long-term intake of calcium above 2,500 milligrams daily has not been studied and should be avoided.

CESAREANS

In 2004, 29.1 percent of all births were C-section deliveries, the highest rate ever reported. A cesarean birth can have both pluses and minuses for breastfeeding mothers. The minuses are that it is major surgery, requires medication, can be quite uncomfortable, and calls for additional recuperation time. A mother in pain may be less able to focus on her new baby. A cesarean birth also means a woman must adjust to her new role as a mother while she recovers from surgery—a double whammy. Mothers who had a C-section delivery need more help and support when they return home.

So what are the pluses? Of course, the big plus is that cesarean birth can save the life of mother and baby. Mothers usually stay in the hospital longer, and for first-time moms this can be a real help. Mothers who leave within twenty-four hours, which is usually the case with vaginal births, won't have the support of the medical staff and the intelligent OB nurses to answer their questions when the baby "wakes up" and really starts to nurse. In this mother's opinion, it is when the milk comes in a few days after delivery that new mothers start to worry about such problems as sore nipples and their ability to breastfeed. Mothers with C-sections may still be in the hospital when this happens and they can get lots of professional assistance and support to help them be more confident about their decision to breastfeed.

A cesarean birth will not impact the timing of milk coming in. If the baby cannot be nursed soon after a cesarean birth, then arrangements should be made for the mother to use a breast pump every three hours until she and her baby can be united.

Mothers who had cesarean births need the same nutrients as any new mother, but probably a few more calories for the first few weeks because of the extra energy required to heal their wounds. Vitamin C and zinc are two nutrients that promote wound healing, so make sure you get a good vitamin C food daily and select some foods such as crabmeat, beef, liver, eggs, chicken, and whole wheat bread for zinc.

Constipation can be a problem after surgery, and some extra high-fiber cereal, whole grain breads, and whole fruits may be helpful. You should also drink enough fluids, which can help with constipation and help prevent a urinary-tract infection (these are more likely after a cesarean birth because a catheter is placed in the bladder during surgery).

POSTPARTUM DEPRESSION

In the first seven days after delivery, 30 to 70 percent of women report feeling the "blues." The blues are a set of symptoms characterized by sadness and fluctuating emotions. These symptoms are probably a very real by-product caused by changing hormones, stress, and sleep deprivation. Postpartum depression is more than the "blues." Approximately 13 percent of new mothers will experience postpartum depression beginning about four weeks to three months after delivery. Women with postpartum depression may experience a depressed mood, sleep disturbances, and changes in appetite, energy, and ability to concentrate. The sooner postpartum depression is identified, the sooner it can be treated. Discuss any concerns you may have with your doctor. If you think about hurting yourself or your baby, get help immediately. There can be physical causes of depression, too, which is why a medical assessment is so important. About 4 to 7 percent of women have a thyroid disorder in the first year postpartum. Such a condition can be linked with postpartum depression, and your doctor can easily conduct a health screen if you tell him your symptoms.

CHOLESTEROL

In the late 1980s, the National Heart, Lung and Blood Institute (NHLBI) started an all-out campaign to bring cholesterol to our attention. The latest report issued in 2001 reconfirms the importance of cholesterol, specifically low-density lipoprotein (LDL)–cholesterol, in preventing heart disease. As a result of these reports, our cholesterol levels are routinely measured during physicals, and much of America is trying to follow a diet that is lower in cholesterol. Many breastfeeding mothers have questions about cholesterol. For instance, can a mother safely adhere to a low-cholesterol diet while breastfeeding? Should a mother restrict cholesterol while breastfeeding? Can her diet affect the cholesterol in her breast milk and hurt or improve her baby's own cholesterol level?

Cholesterol is a fatlike substance that we make in our liver and consume in food. It is present in every body tissue. Only animal foods contain cholesterol; fruits, vegetables, and grains are cholesterol free. Cholesterol is now considered unhealthy, but that's not true. We need cholesterol. It makes up part of some essential hormones and tissues. What *is* harmful is an excessive blood level of the stuff. When blood cholesterol levels are too high, the risk for heart disease is thought to increase.

Naturally, researchers and mothers would like to know just

how to start infants off on the right dietary path to avoid a cholesterol problem in adulthood. Though the subject has been studied quite a bit, the answers are still inconclusive.

Research suggests that a rise in cholesterol level may be a natural part of pregnancy and lactation. In a 1985 Swedish study reported in *Obstetrics and Gynecology*, mothers had higher cholesterol levels eight weeks after they gave birth than they did before conception.

Breastfeeding mothers tend to have higher cholesterol levels than mothers who aren't nursing. In a study conducted by Dr. R. H. Knopp that compared the cholesterol levels of new mothers, the lactating mothers had a mean cholesterol level of 207, whereas the women who were not breastfeeding had a mean cholesterol level of 188. This is a significant difference. A desirable cholesterol level is thought to be less than 200 milligrams per deciliter. A reading between 200 and 239 is said to be borderline high.

In this study, the breastfeeding mothers might have had a total cholesterol level that was technically borderline, but their mean level of "good cholesterol," or high-density lipoprotein (HDL)–cholesterol, was 65; other mothers had a mean HDL-cholesterol of only 51. The more HDL we have in our blood the better, because HDL seems to help carry the "bad cholesterol," or LDL-cholesterol, out of our bodies. In this study, the levels of HDL were in the healthy range for both the nursing and the bottle-feeding mothers, but it's nice to know that the breastfeeding moms had a higher level of HDL, which many nutritionists think protects against atherosclerosis, or clogged arteries. In fact, a 2004 study from researchers in London found that preterm infants who had been breastfed had better cholesterol levels when they became adolescents, potentially decreasing their lifetime risk of heart disease.

The cholesterol content of your milk will stay remarkably constant in the range of 100 to 150 milligrams per liter of milk no matter what you eat. This is true even if you have a very high level of blood cholesterol yourself. You wouldn't want to decrease the cholesterol in your baby's milk anyway. Cholesterol is essential to the newborn. She needs it for proper brain development and for the protection of nerve cells.

While a mother's diet won't influence the cholesterol level in her breast milk, it can affect the milk's fatty-acid content. For example, when mothers eat a diet rich in polyunsaturated fats like vegetable and corn oil, their milk content of linoleic acid can almost double. Dr. Margot Mellies found this change in the fatty-acid composition of breast milk when she studied fourteen breastfeeding mothers and their infants in the late 1970s. Linoleic acid is an essential fatty acid that is particularly important to the growth and development of infants. So the type of fat we eat can affect the fats in breast milk even though it doesn't affect the milk's cholesterol content.

The current recommendation for adults is that we eat no more than 300 milligrams of cholesterol per day and that our fat intake be approximately 30 percent of our total calories, with not more than 10 percent of that fat from saturated fats. Read labels, keep your saturated fat intake low—below 25 grams, probably closer to 20 grams—and avoid *trans*-fats. *Trans*-fat is another type of fat that can raise blood cholesterol levels. The meal plan in chapter 6 meets these goals. You'll benefit from following these prudent guidelines while breastfeeding and from continuing them for the rest of your life.

Mothers who have high cholesterol levels should consult a registered dietitian for specific counseling. Mothers who must follow a low-cholesterol diet while breastfeeding can switch to 1 percent milk, choose low-fat cheese, trim fat from meats, avoid fried foods, and eat lots of fruits, vegetables, and grains without gobs of butter or rich sauces. Mothers don't need to eliminate eggs, meat, or milk entirely to control cholesterol. Fish-oil supplements, which are rich in the essential fatty acid docosahexaenoic acid, or DHA, have for some time been popular among individuals who want to reduce their risk of heart disease. The oil is thought to reduce the risk of heart disease by lowering triglyceride levels and reducing the tendency of the blood to clot.

Triglycerides are made from the extra calories we eat that are not needed right away and get stored as triglyceride. Between meals, the body releases triglyceride from the fat we store. Fish lowers triglyceride levels and Eskimos who eat fish as a dietary staple have much less heart disease than most other people.

In the mid-1980s, Dr. William Harris asked eight breastfeeding mothers to participate in a study of fish-oil supplements. This study was designed to see if by increasing their dietary intake of DHA, mothers could also increase the level of DHA in their breast milk. DHA is abundant in the human brain and eye. Your baby incorporates DHA into her nerve tissues while in the womb and during the first year of her life.

The eight mothers took fish-oil supplements rich in DHA for up to twenty-eight days. The supplements were the equivalent of eating ten to twenty-three ounces of cod or sole, or three ounces of salmon or mackerel daily. All the mothers significantly increased the levels of DHA in their breast milk. Their babies were getting more DHA, which could have a positive effect on their eye and brain development. Dr. S. R. Cheruku, another researcher writing in the *American Journal of Clinical Nutrition,* found that infants whose mothers had a high intake of DHA had better sleep patterns, possibly because the DHA has a positive connection with neurological development. Historically, infant formula has not contained DHA whereas breast milk always has. Many formula companies now add DHA to their formula in an attempt to replicate the DHA found naturally in breast milk. Breastfeeding mothers will want to include some fish in their diet. Read about fish safety on page 145.

VEGETARIAN DIETS

Some vegetarians simply avoid red meat like beef, lamb, and pork, while others eliminate all animal foods from their diets. It is only at the very strict end of the spectrum, when all meat, milk, poultry, and eggs are eliminated, that vegetarian mothers and babies risk deficiency.

Cases of malnutrition in breastfed babies have occurred when vegetarian mothers eat extremely restricted diets. In one case, a six-month-old infant was admitted to the University of California Medical Center in San Diego in a coma. He was born apparently healthy to a mother who had consumed no vitamin B_{12} foods such as meat, eggs, or milk for eight years before her pregnancy. The mother had no symptoms of B_{12} deficiency, and her breastfed baby appeared to develop normally until about four months of age, at which time his development started to regress; he became lethargic and irritable, and bruised easily. It is important to note that this little baby had a B_{12} deficiency even though his mother was symptom free. I'm happy to report that the baby improved dramatically within just four days of treatment with B_{12} and was discharged from the hospital after fourteen days, with a prescription for a daily vitamin B_{12} supplement in his mom's hand.

This is an extreme case. Most vegetarian mothers are knowledgeable and careful about what they eat, and aware that vitamin B_{12} and vitamin D are crucial to their babies' health. It is only those mothers who are very strict vegetarians who must be cautioned about extreme B_{12} deficiency.

Parents who are vegetarian often want to raise a vegetarian child. This can be safe if the child's diet is planned carefully. A vegetarian child is at a greater risk for nutritional inadequacies than a vegetarian adult. The reason for this is that babies and young children need lots of calories and nutrients. A diet high in vegetables and grains is very bulky and can fill a child up before he has met his protein, calorie, and vitamin needs. An egg provides 70 calories, lots of protein, and many nutrients in one ounce of digestible food. To get the same amount of protein, your child would have to eat one or two cups of rice and beans. You can see the problem.

Vegetarian breastfeeding moms must eat enough calories, at least 1,800 to 2,700 calories every day. Calories are essential so the protein in the diet can be used for building and repairing instead of being burned as fuel. Calories can come from every food. Protein can be found in dairy foods, egg, soy milk, soy products, beans, and grains. Despite the elimination of red meat, vegetarians are not routinely iron-deficient, perhaps because vitamin C, which enhances iron absorption and is abundant in fruits and vegetables, reduces the risk.

Breastfeeding vegan mothers—women who exclude meat, poultry, eggs, seafood, milk products, and honey—have very special nutrition considerations. Vitamin B_{12}, vitamin D, and the omega-3 fatty acids (typically found in fish) are all inadequate in the vegan diet. A B_{12} supplement of 2.6 mcg is essential and a vitamin D supplement is required unless there is adequate sun exposure of fifteen to thirty minutes daily. DHA, an omega-3 fatty acid, is abundant in fish and DHA supplements made from algae, but flaxseed oil, walnuts, canola oil, soybean oil, and tofu carry alpha-linolenic acid (ALA), which can be converted to DHA. Although how much ALA is converted to DHA is unknown, these foods should be included in the vegan diet.

NURSING YOUR PREMATURE BABY

Babies born early can definitely benefit from their mothers' breast milk. With support from the medical staff and from their families, mothers with premature babies can successfully nurse their infants.

Mothers of premature babies often have to wait before they can be united with their little ones. Sometimes this separation may be brief, and if the child is strong and can suck, he may be able to nurse quite soon after he is born. But many mothers are separated from their infants for an extended period and must spend their first days and sometimes weeks using a breast pump. This takes tremendous commitment, but nursing your baby, even if it means pumping and storing breast milk, will be tremendously rewarding. Your baby gets the benefit of your healthful breast milk, and you'll get to feel that you're really participating in your baby's care.

Mothers who have premature babies produce preterm milk that is richer in protein, sodium, and chloride than the milk of mothers with full-term babies. These extra nutrients are essential to meeting a preemie's needs.

Make sure to let your doctor know that you want to breast-feed. A lactation consultant can be a tremendous help to the mother of a premature baby. Your doctor may be affiliated with a lactation consultant; if not, check the Resources section for suggestions on finding a consultant in your area. Check the Resources section, too, if you need help finding a breast pump.

If you are discharged from the hospital before your baby, try to rest and eat well. This will keep up your milk production and help you maintain your own health. If you must be at the hospital for long periods, bring some good, healthy snacks and ask if there is a spot where you can sit down and put your feet up between feedings. This is a stressful time for you and your family, so pay extra attention to taking good care of yourself.

Good Snacks to Bring to the Hospital

Yogurt in individual containers
Peanut butter and crackers
Juice boxes or cans
Sliced cheese and bread
Whole, ready-to-eat fruit like peaches, pears, and apples
Ready-to-eat sandwiches

FEEDING THE MOTHER OF TWINS OR TRIPLETS

Common sense alone is going to tell you that the mother of twins or triplets is going to need more food than the mother of a single child. Your body will secrete about 420 to 700 calories a day for each child who is being exclusively breastfed, which means that you need an extra 500 calories for each baby being nursed. The good news is that your breasts can meet this demand. Studies show that while most babies drink only 500 to 700 grams of milk daily, a mother can make 2,000 to 3,000 grams if the demand is there. In the 1600s a wet nurse could feed six infants daily. It is not milk supply that is the issue but time and having only two hands. Mothers with multiple children need to ask for help.

TANDEM NURSING

Mothers who conceive before the first nursing child is weaned and then go on to tandem-nurse have special needs. The demand for all the nutrients will increase because the mother needs enough nutrition to nourish her pregnancy and to keep up an adequate supply of breast milk without depleting her own reserves. There have been no nutritional studies that identify particular problems of tandem nursing, but these mothers should plan to get the special nutrients needed for lactation (calcium and zinc) plus those needed for a healthy pregnancy (iron, folic acid, and protein). Adequate weight gain is an important issue. The mom who is tandem nursing doesn't have much room for junk food.

Once the new baby is born, the mother's milk returns first to colostrum and then to the early postpartum milk. The younger infant should nurse first and feed until satisfied. (Usually older children nurse for comfort, not nutrition.) The older child can nurse after the baby is done. Find the book *Adventures in Tandem Nursing: Breastfeeding During Pregnancy and Beyond* by Hillary Flower (La Leche League, 2003).

DIABETES AND BREASTFEEDING

Today more and more mothers who have diabetes are delivering happy, healthy babies, and these mothers with preexisting and gestational diabetes are being encouraged to breastfeed. Diabetes is greatly affected by diet. A breastfeeding mother who has diabetes must eat a balanced diet that is divided into many small meals. These frequent small meals help keep her blood sugar stable.

There are several types of diabetes: gestational, insulin dependent, and non–insulin dependent. Mothers who develop gestational diabetes while pregnant often find that it disappears after they give birth. The rise in blood sugar is caused by the stress the baby causes while growing in the womb. After the mother delivers, blood sugar probably returns to normal, and the breast milk is not affected. Women who develop gestational diabetes have an increased incidence of non–insulin-dependent diabetes when they get older. In fact, 50 to 60 percent of women with gestational diabetes develop permanent diabetes later in life. Most women can reduce their risk of diabetes through a healthy lifestyle, which includes regular exercise and weight control. If you have gestational diabetes, you, too, can reduce your risk of permanent diabetes or delay its development by keeping your weight in the ideal range and by exercising regularly. (See chapter 7 for more information.) A recent study in the *Journal of the American Medical Association* found that lactation itself may offer protection against diabetes. The study looked at the rate of diabetes in breastfeeding women in the ongoing Nurses Health Study conducted through the Brigham and Women's Hospital in Boston. There was a lower incidence of diabetes mellitus among the women who had breastfed their babies.

Mothers with insulin-dependent and non–insulin-dependent diabetes will want to pay careful attention to what they eat throughout their pregnancy and while breastfeeding. The information given here is only a guideline. Every mother with diabetes should consult a registered dietitian or diabetes educator for specific nutrition recommendations that are coordinated with her physician's care plan. Women with diabetes walk a tightrope. The goal is to prevent high blood sugar while avoiding low blood sugar. It is not uncommon for mothers who take insulin (the hormone that regulates blood sugar) to find that the amount of insulin they need decreases while they breastfeed. That's because some of the sugar that would normally circulate in the mother's blood is now being used to make up part of her milk supply. These mothers will need less insulin and their blood-sugar levels will be lower.

Very low blood sugar, or hypoglycemia, is of course undesirable. Its symptoms include weakness, dizziness, headaches, and possibly even blackouts. Hypoglycemia can inhibit your milk production. To prevent hypoglycemia, eat meals at prescribed times, eat more if you exercise, and always carry a quick-acting carbohydrate like sugar packets or glucose tablets. Some nursing diabetic mothers find that they need to decrease their evening dose of insulin to prevent hypoglycemia.

The calorie recommendations in chapter 6 can also be used by the mother with diabetes. Be aware that methods to determine calories are only approximate, and adjustments need to be made based on weight, hunger, activity, and overall satisfaction. The 2004 Diabetes Care guidelines suggest that breastfeeding mothers may meet their needs on as little as 1,800 calories daily. A mother who has diabetes and who takes insulin should not go for more than three hours without something to eat. If she does, she risks developing low blood sugar. If you find you overeat by consuming half your recommended calories in one sitting, your blood sugar may rise too high. A gentle walk may help lower your sugar level.

The diabetic diet often begins with about 50 percent of total calories as carbohydrate. Carbohydrate foods include foods in the bread, milk, and fruit groups. Women may need a carbohydrate-containing snack before and during breastfeeding to keep blood sugar stable.

Mothers with diabetes who choose to breastfeed will be happy to learn that breastfeeding may protect their babies from developing the disease; studies repeatedly demonstrate the protective effect of breast milk. One of the greatest obstacles for mothers with diabetes is that their newborns are given an examination soon after birth and might not be put to the breast immediately after delivery. The sooner the baby is put to the breast, the more likely the mother and baby will be successful at breastfeeding. Before you deliver, tell your doctor that you want to breastfeed. If she expects a long delay before you can nurse your child, ask if you can use a breast pump in the interim to stimulate your milk production. Because diabetes increases the risk of body infection, breastfeeding moms with diabetes must not ignore sore, cracked nipples or signs of mastitis. Call your health care provider if you suspect any type of infection in your breasts.

IRON-DEFICIENCY ANEMIA

Approximately 15 percent of women of childbearing age have iron-deficiency anemia. Iron is part of the hemoglobin in your blood, which carries oxygen to your cells. Iron-deficiency anemia occurs when your body's stores of iron are depleted. Symptoms include fatigue, weakness, shortness of breath, and pallor. Your iron stores won't be depleted if you skip a meal or don't eat iron-rich foods for a day or two. In most cases, it takes a long time to deplete iron stores. Women are at greater risk for iron deficiency than men because menstruation causes monthly loss of blood and iron. During pregnancy, a woman's blood volume increases, and her developing placenta and baby require iron, too, which can further deplete the mother's stores.

The DRI for iron for pregnant women is set at 27 milligrams. For breastfeeding mothers, it drops down to 9 to 10 milligrams. Breastfeeding doesn't draw much iron; a mother secretes less than 1 milligram of iron in a day's supply of breast milk. Less iron is needed while breastfeeding than when you have your period. Since in many cases your period won't resume for several months while you nurse, breastfeeding actually gives you an opportunity to conserve iron, and it's a good idea for women who are iron deficient. But if your period starts again while you are breastfeeding, your demand for iron will increase, so make sure you get some very good sources.

Iron can be a tough nutrient to get, particularly for women on calorie-restricted diets or women who don't eat animal foods such as beef, lamb, and so on, which are the best iron sources. The iron that is available from vegetables is less absorbable than the iron in meat. Milk is also a very poor source of iron.

If iron deficiency is a problem for you, try to eat iron-rich foods (a complete listing of these foods is given in chapter 3). There are other things you can try to enhance iron absorption:

- Eat a food rich in vitamin C with every meal—it will enhance absorption of the iron you eat. Drink orange juice, eat a citrus fruit for dessert, or eat a vitamin C–rich vegetable, such as tomatoes or broccoli.
- Eat a small amount of meat with every meal.
- Eat iron-fortified cereals, bread, and pasta.
- Cook in cast-iron pots. Studies show that some of the iron passes from the pot into your food and can become a significant source of iron.
- Studies have found that tea and coffee can inhibit iron absorption, so drink these an hour before or after you eat your meal.
- Ask your doctor for an iron supplement. Unfortunately, the iron consumed in tablet form isn't nearly as well absorbed as that from real food. Iron supplements can also be constipating and upsetting to the stomach.

Even if you have iron-deficiency anemia, your baby won't be affected when you breastfeed. The iron content of breast milk is not affected by your diet or the level of iron in your blood. Iron-deficiency anemia is quite uncommon in breastfed babies under six months old. Your little one was born with a six-month supply of iron, even if your intake of iron while pregnant was less than ideal; this supply helps ensure adequate iron levels. The exception to this rule has been seen in breastfed babies who are given solid food early, say at the three-month mark. Early solids can decrease a baby's intake of breast milk, which contains a small but highly absorbable form of iron. Babies who start on solid foods early should be fed iron-rich foods. Iron-fortified cereal can be a good choice.

Infants exclusively fed breast milk beyond age six months were not found to be anemic, but infants breastfed for less than six months were at greater risk of iron-deficiency anemia specifically if they did not get a food source rich in iron.

HIGH BLOOD PRESSURE

High blood pressure gives no early warning signs. Untreated, it can cause headaches, kidney disease, even stroke. If you've had high blood pressure, make sure you get regular follow-up care. Routine blood pressure readings are the only way to know if you have the disease under control.

Women with high blood pressure can breastfeed. Women who are on medications will need to discuss with their doctors the fact that they are breastfeeding. You may want to talk with both the doctor who is prescribing your medication and your baby's pediatrician. Breastfeeding may actually lower a woman's blood pressure. It serves as a diuretic, pulling extra fluid into the breast milk. The higher levels of prolactin that are present in breastfeeding women may also help lower blood pressure. You may be concerned about what to eat to control your high blood pressure while you breastfeed, but you should meet your needs for feeding the baby first. You'll be glad to hear that the same diet that is healthy for breastfeeding moms can also help control high blood pressure.

Many people are aware that salt has been linked with high blood pressure in some individuals. In these cases, reducing sodium intake can lower blood pressure. Breastfeeding moms can cut back on salt by simply putting away the salt shaker and avoiding foods that are obviously salty.

The upper intake for sodium has been set at 2,300 milligrams. Women need a bit more sodium while breastfeeding (about 135 milligrams more), but because studies have found that the standard American diet provides 1,800 to 5,000 milligrams of sodium a day, you can see that getting too much sodium is more a concern than getting too little. By not adding salt to food while cooking or at the table and by avoiding obviously salty foods, you can easily reduce sodium intake to 2,000 to 4,000 milligrams a day.

There are four lifestyle practices that have a significant impact on blood pressure. They include weight control, salt intake, moderate alcohol intake, and regular exercise. Calcium, potassium, and magnesium can all have an effect on hypertension.

- Calcium—Calcium has been found to have an antihypertensive effect in some individuals.
- Potassium—This mineral may lower blood pressure by depleting sodium in the blood. Good food sources of potassium include all fresh fruits and vegetables. Moms should get at least two servings of each daily. Fresh meat and poultry are good sources, too.
- Magnesium—Individuals with high blood pressure were able to lower blood pressure by increasing magnesium intake, according to one research study. Breastfeeding moms are encouraged to get adequate magnesium from food, including green leafy vegetables, whole grains, nuts, meat, and beans.
- Calories—Reaching and maintaining ideal body weight can be extremely effective for controlling high blood pressure. A 5 percent weight loss alone has been found to lower blood pressure and in some cases eliminate the need for medication.
- Alcohol—One percent of American women have high blood

pressure because of the amount of alcohol they drink. Women who choose to breastfeed should follow the recommended restrictions on alcohol to prevent this from being a problem.

Please note that supplements are not the recommended way to obtain these nutrients. Food is your best source for them all. The Dietary Approach to Stop Hypertension (DASH) Diet incorporates all these nutrients in its eating plans. Learn more at www.nhlbi.nih.gov and search "DASH Diet."

HEMORRHOIDS AND CONSTIPATION

If you have the misfortune of developing these two conditions together, you're going to be uncomfortable. Constipation is technically defined as not having a bowel movement for three days. (In case you didn't know, you don't have to have a daily bowel movement.) If constipation is a problem, look at what you're eating. Foods rich in fiber—fruit, vegetables, and whole grain bread and cereals—are your friends. (If your diet has been low in fiber, start high-fiber foods slowly; too much all at once might make you uncomfortable.) Raisins, prunes, and figs can be helpful, too. Fluids help keep stools soft and prevent constipation, so remember to drink plenty of fluids—the latest recommendation is nine cups daily. The fluid in coffee, tea, soft drinks, fruit, juice, pudding, even yogurt can all contribute to the nine-cup recommendation.

Most doctors won't recommend a laxative except on a temporary basis. Regular use can become habit-forming, eventually making a bowel movement without a laxative impossible. If constipation is a problem, allow yourself the time to go to the bathroom. That advice might have sounded ridiculous before you had a baby, but as a new mom you might be able to see the problem. Many moms are too busy to allow themselves a few personal moments, and for them constipation can become quite a problem.

If you developed or aggravated hemorrhoids while pregnant, you're not alone. Because of the increased pressure on the anal opening, lots of pregnant women develop hemorrhoids. Hemorrhoids usually aren't dangerous, but they can become a painful problem if you're constipated, so try to avoid constipation by eating lots of fiber-rich foods. If you have painful hemorrhoids, consult your doctor about medical treatment.

High-Fiber Foods

Cereals: All-Bran, Bran Buds, 100% Bran flakes, unprocessed raw bran, Shredded Wheat.

Whole Grains: Brown rice, cracked wheat, bulgur, kasha.

Bread: 100% whole wheat products (sliced bread, pita bread, bagels, English muffins), bran bread, rye bread, Bran'nola pumpernickel. (Always check labels if you're looking for whole grains. The first ingredient should say whole wheat. Wheat flour can mean white flour, and this isn't high in fiber.)

Crackers: Any cracker listing whole wheat as the first ingredient, graham crackers, Ry-Krisp.

Beans and peas: Lentils, kidney beans, chickpeas, baked beans.

Seeds and nuts: Sesame, sunflower, pumpkin, and poppy seeds, peanuts with skins, almonds with skins, walnuts, cashews.

Fruit: Apples, grapefruit, grapes, berries, mangoes, melons, oranges, pears, and peaches. Wash well or buy organic and leave the peel on.

Vegetables: All kinds. Wash well and peel waxed cucumbers and peppers.

MOM GOES BACK TO WORK

Rejoining the workforce is not a health issue like diabetes or high blood pressure, but it does present unique problems for the nursing mother. Without planning or support by family, friends, employers, and coworkers, a new mother can easily become overwhelmed and overstressed.

Mothers who work outside the home are more likely than others to choose breastfeeding at first, but they are apt to wean sooner or add supplemental bottles. Surveys show that fatigue, difficulty with pumping and milk storage, concerns about adequate milk production, having enough time for work, and even enough time to eat are a mother's top concerns when she goes back to her job.

In a study on the working mother and breastfeeding published in the *Journal of Public Health Policy,* six barriers to continued breastfeeding were identified:

1. Lack of good child care near or at the mother's work site.
2. No place for a mother to nurse, pump, or store milk.
3. Inadequate employment policies regarding maternity leave and job security.
4. Disapproving attitudes regarding breastfeeding by employers and coworkers.
5. Lack of knowledge about breastfeeding on the mother's part.
6. Lack of knowledge about breastfeeding on the part of health care workers, particularly those involved with employee health.

Being well informed about the hurdles you may face when returning to work is probably your best defense against problems. To make your transition easier, try the following:

- Before you deliver, try to seek out other mothers at your work site to see how they coped.
- Find another mother—a friend, a coworker, or a La Leche League member—to give you firsthand practical advice and support. Lactation consultants can also be real lifesavers.
- Ask your family for help. Having people run errands, prepare

some casseroles, or perhaps pick up your baby at the sitter's may make your life easier.

- Consider working part-time or trying to do some work at home. Some lucky moms can job-share, with two people working half of the same job, allowing more time for each to be at home.
- Try to find a child care situation that's close to work so you can feed your baby during breaks.

While you cope with working and caring for a new baby, remember that breastfeeding doesn't go on forever. When your baby is very little, it may seem as though the situation is hopeless and overwhelming. It may give you comfort to remember that it's all temporary. Soon enough—and it may even seem like it's too soon—your baby won't be completely dependent on just you.

GOOD FOODS FOR BUSY MOMS

Eating well while working can be a real challenge. A working mother has to take care of her baby (a full-time job in itself) in addition to her job and household responsibilities. Lots of women put their baby first and leave little time for their own needs. Eating well is important for you *and* the baby. If you don't eat enough, you'll feel even more fatigued and run down.

The best foods are the ones you make from scratch, but I would rather see a mother eat a frozen dinner than skip a meal. Here is a list of healthy ready-to-eat foods that might work for you when you're rushed at work.

- Yogurt or yogurt drink with 30 percent calcium or more per serving.
- Ready-made sandwiches from the deli or supermarket.
- Frozen dinners (if you have a microwave at work).

- Crackers and a jar of peanut butter (you can keep these in your desk).
- Fresh fruit—apples, bananas, pears.
- Nuts—limit to ¼-cup portion per snack.
- Dried fruits—be aware of the caloric content; read the label.
- Individual packs of applesauce, fruits, or pudding.

10

EAT WELL, FEEL WELL

Most of your usual recipes can be part of your menu while you're breastfeeding. Some women feel that certain spices, seasonings, or vegetables bother the baby. This is a very individual matter. If you feel some of my ingredients are too strong, just cut back on the amounts I suggest.

You'll be an unusual new mother if you have the time or the desire to do a lot of cooking. But you must feed yourself, and if you make healthy, satisfying foods, you'll feel better and so will your baby. Make double portions of recipes and use your freezer to keep ready-to-eat foods on hand.

A NEW DAY IN THE KITCHEN

For many families, a child brings renewed interest in healthy eating. It's not uncommon for people to become more responsible about what they eat once they become parents. Breastfeeding mothers in particular are very conscientious about what they eat. Here's a list of cooking tips that will help your whole family eat more healthily:

- Try reducing the fat content in your favorite recipe by half. For example, if you make a chicken stew that calls for four tablespoons of olive oil, simply reduce it to two. No one will notice the difference. (In most cases you can't reduce the fat in baked goods without altering the recipe.)

- Try using water or cooking wine to sauté in instead of butter or oil.
- Spray a pan with oil to prevent sticking and add just 1 to 2 teaspoons of cooking oil for flavor.
- If you're using convenience foods like boxed macaroni and cheese or rice mixes, cut the amount of butter or margarine called for in the directions by one-half.
- Use skim or 1 percent milk in any recipe calling for milk.
- Buy and use low-fat cheeses, or use smaller amounts of a strong-flavored cheese like Romano or Parmesan to substitute for high-fat hard cheeses.
- Use canned evaporated skim milk to replace cream in recipes such as cream soups.
- Try substituting low-fat yogurt for sour cream in recipes. This can work in baked goods such as coffee cake as well as in a Stroganoff dish (keep in mind that yogurt can become a bit runny in a sautéed dish).
- If a recipe calls for a half cup of vegetables, try doubling (or tripling) that amount to increase your vegetable intake.
- Mix low-fat yogurt with mayonnaise in such things as potato salad or macaroni salad or when preparing tuna salad. This also works great on green salads—top a large tossed salad with one tablespoon creamy dressing mixed with two tablespoons low-fat plain yogurt.
- Trim all visible fat from meats and bake or broil instead of frying. Regular hamburger can be as low in fat as the more expensive lean choices, depending on how you cook it. If you use it in a meat loaf and the fat is kept trapped in the pan, then it will be high in fat. If you broil a hamburger on a pan that allows the fat to drip away, then it will be just as low in fat as the lean burger.
- Try substituting ground turkey for ground beef in recipes.

- Trim the skin from poultry.
- When making soups or gravies, refrigerate and later remove the fat that rises to the surface.
- Sprinkle confectioners' sugar on cake instead of high-fat frosting.

Cooking can destroy nutrients. To get the most out of the food you buy, try the following:

- Keep ripe fruits and vegetables cold.
- Cook vegetables for as short a time as possible and with as little water as possible.
- Don't pare or trim vegetables excessively—the leaves on broccoli stems, for instance, are very nutritious. Do peel waxed produce. Don't wash or soak vegetables for prolonged periods.
- Avoid boiling vegetables.

START YOUR DAY OFF RIGHT

A good breakfast is essential to maintaining your energy, especially while you're breastfeeding. Even if you weren't a breakfast eater in the past, you should feel hungrier now and should want to eat breakfast. You don't have to eat eggs and sausage. A morning meal of fruit, cereal with milk or yogurt, toast, juice, and a cup of coffee will give you protein, calcium, and carbohydrates and a good start on your day's nutrients. You can divide that into two small mini–morning meals, too.

A good breakfast should provide 20 to 25 percent of your calories (that's about 540 to 675 calories). Many mothers will feel better if they include some protein at breakfast to carry them through the morning. This might be cheese, milk, peanut butter, yogurt, cooked fish, eggs, ham, or beans.

TEN NO-FUSS BREAKFAST IDEAS

Some of these meals can be put together the night before. Our house is always busy in the morning, so having food ready to heat helps reduce the morning frazzles.

1. Cereal with milk and fruit.
2. Baked eggs. Mix 2 eggs with 1 tablespoon of milk and, if you wish, 1 tablespoon grated cheese and 2 tablespoons chopped tomato. Put together the night before. Bake at 375°F for fifteen minutes or until firm, or microwave for two minutes on high, stir and cook one minute more, and let rest one minute, covered, before serving.
3. Oatmeal with milk and fruit. Mix ¼ cup oatmeal with ¼ cup milk plus ¼ cup water and let stand overnight. Cook per instructions in the microwave or on the stove, and then top with fresh fruit.
4. Grandma's Early Morning Coffee Cake with a dish of yogurt and fresh fruit (see page 182 for recipe).
5. Frozen waffles (try the whole wheat waffles at least once) topped with yogurt and fresh fruit—skip the butter.
6. Poached egg on an English muffin.
7. Half a bagel topped with cottage cheese, sliced tomato, red onion, and black pepper (the onion and pepper are optional). The sliced tomato is an excellent source of vitamin C.
8. Breakfast fruit shake. Put 1 cup yogurt and 1 cup canned or fresh fruit (seeded and peeled) in the blender the night before. Mix in the morning. Enjoy a few slices of toast along with it.
9. Cook a turkey sausage patty or Canadian bacon instead of pork sausage. Serve with sliced tomato, whole wheat toast, milk, and a slice of fruit.
10. Peanut butter on whole wheat toast with sliced bananas.

Breakfast at the Drive-Thru

No one likes to admit they do it, but breakfast on the run is not uncommon. Good choices can be made; consider calories, choose something with protein, and try to get some fruit. Most fruit will come in the form of juice, but a whole fruit like a banana is likely to be more sustaining (you might want to bring one with you from home).

Food	Calories
Sesame bagel, plain	455
Cream cheese, 4 tablespoons	204
Hotcakes, three	340
Maple syrup, ¼ cup	208
Egg and cheese and ham on an English muffin	275
Hash browns	130
Fruit yogurt parfait	155
Orange juice, 12 ounces	140
Coffee cake muffin	710
Doughnut	200–330
Coffee, black	0
Coffee coolatta, with cream	370

Start Your Day with Zinc

While you're nursing, you need to eat about 12 to 14 milligrams of zinc every day. A cereal rich in zinc is a great way to help meet that requirement. The zinc content of selected cereals is listed below. Not all the zinc you eat in food will actually get absorbed, which makes it extra important for you to select zinc-rich foods.

Cereal	Zinc in 1-Cup Serving (mg)
All-Bran	11.1
Apple Jacks	3.7

Bran Buds	11.1
Cap'n Crunch	4.01
Nutri-Grain cereals (all varieties)	more than 5.3
100% Bran	5.74
Special K	2.77
Wheat germ	18.9*

*Great source of zinc, but it contains 432 calories and 12 grams of fat.

RECIPES FOR HEALTHY LIVING

Now that you know good nutrition is important while breast-feeding, here are some recipes that combine good taste with good nutrition. I have tried to keep the preparation time quick and the ingredient lists short. To help you use the menu-planning system from chapter 6, I've included the approximate number of portions from each food group that the recipes provide.

Home-Baked Breakfasts
Eating a good breakfast is the best way to start your day. Whole grain cereal, fresh fruit, and milk or yogurt is a simple and nutritious start. When you feel like baking and have the time, try one of the recipes that follow.

GRANDMA'S EARLY MORNING COFFEE CAKE

When I was a little girl my mother would occasionally treat her brood of four hungry children to this special coffee cake. She assembled it the night before, refrigerated it, then added the topping and baked it while our family got dressed and ready for school. She made it again when she came to help me out when my girls were born, and it brought back fond memories of warm family breakfasts. I hope you enjoy it!

Cake	Topping
3 tablespoons butter	2 tablespoons wheat germ
½ cup sugar	3 tablespoons sugar
1 egg, beaten	3 tablespoons melted butter
1 cup milk	¾ teaspoon cinnamon
1 teaspoon vanilla extract	5 tablespoons crushed corn flakes
1½ cups flour	
2 teaspoons baking powder	
¼ teaspoon salt	
⅔ cup wheat germ	

Preheat the oven to 375°F. Grease an 8-inch square or round cake pan. Cream the butter with the sugar. Add the egg, milk, and vanilla extract. Then add the dry ingredients and blend well. Pour the batter into pan. Mix the topping ingredients together and sprinkle over the batter. Bake for 25 to 30 minutes, or until it tests done with a cake tester.

TO MAKE AHEAD: Mix the cake; pour into the pan; mix the topping but do not sprinkle it on the cake. Refrigerate covered. Before baking, add the topping.

Makes nine portions; 1 starch and 1 fat per serving.

WHOLE WHEAT AND BRAN MUFFINS

These muffins taste good and provide lots of fiber and zinc. Of course they're easy to make, too.

¾ cup wheat bran	2 teaspoons grated orange or
¾ cup whole wheat flour	lemon peel (use organic or
½ cup Bran Buds	unwaxed fruit)
½ cup brown sugar	1 egg, lightly beaten
2 teaspoons baking soda	⅔ cup plain yogurt
¼ teaspoon salt	¼ cup vegetable oil

Preheat the oven to 400°F. Mix all the dry ingredients, including the grated peel. In a separate large bowl, mix the egg, yogurt, and oil and blend well. Fold in the dry ingredients until just blended—don't overbeat. The batter will be thick and grainy-looking. Pour it into lightly oiled muffin tins and bake for 18 to 20 minutes.

Makes twelve muffins; 1 starch and 1 fat per muffin.

VARIATIONS: To make blueberry or raisin muffins, fold in 1 cup of blueberries or ½ cup of raisins to the finished batter and cook as directed.

Main Dish Winners

The recipes that follow are designed to be low in fat, high in flavor. Ingredients should be readily available in your market and the recipes easy to assemble. Enjoy!

CREAMY PASTA PRIMAVERA

Years ago when my husband and I decided to eat less fat, we developed this recipe for a rich, creamy pasta. When I became a new mother, I really liked this recipe because it was fast, healthy, and a great way to get more calcium.

½ pound pasta
1 clove garlic, chopped
1 tablespoon olive oil
2 carrots, scrubbed and diced
1 cup fresh or frozen green
vegetables (broccoli, peas, green
beans, zucchini)

1 cup plain, low-fat yogurt
1 cup low-fat cottage cheese
2 tablespoons grated Parmesan
cheese

Bring a large pot of water to boil for the pasta. In a large frying pan, sauté the garlic in oil; add the raw carrots (and raw green vegetables if you're using them). Cover and let simmer on the lowest heat about 5 minutes, then remove from heat. If using a frozen green vegetable, add it in the last minute of cooking. The vegetables should be tender but not mushy.

Add the pasta to the boiling water and cook according to the package directions. Meanwhile, blend the yogurt, cottage cheese, and Parmesan cheese in a blender until creamy and smooth. Drain the pasta. Toss with the yogurt-cheese sauce and three-quarters of the cooked vegetables. Arrange on serving dish and sprinkle with remaining vegetables. Serve hot with extra grated cheese, bread, and a good salad.

Makes four good-size portions; 4 starch, ¼ milk, 1 fat, 1 protein, and 1½ vegetable per serving.

YOGURT FRIED CHICKEN

Fried chicken went off our menu years ago, but I miss the crispy texture. This recipe is a terrific way to get the taste of fried food and lots of protein and calcium without all the fat. If you shy away from cooking with yogurt, try this at least once. It does not have a sour yogurt taste.

8 chicken thighs (use another cut if you prefer)	*1 cup seasoned bread crumbs*
2 cups plain yogurt	*2 teaspoons olive oil*

Preheat the oven to 375°F. Remove the skin from the chicken and roll the chicken in yogurt, coating the chicken liberally. Then roll it in the seasoned bread crumbs. Place the coated chicken on a lightly oiled baking dish. Drizzle with the olive oil and bake for 45 minutes.

Makes four portions; 1 starch, ½ milk, and 4 protein per serving.

PASTA WITH FISH SAUCE

Lots of people don't eat fish because they think it smells or don't know how to cook it. Please try this dish even if you aren't a fish lover. It's easy and oh so good!

1 pound cut-up white fish such as cod, haddock, halibut, or pollock (frozen will do, but thaw first)	*½ cup white wine* *½ cup water* *1 tablespoon fresh chopped parsley*

¼ teaspoon dried thyme   1 pound pasta
Juice from ½ lemon
1 clove garlic, chopped
2 tablespoons olive oil

Place the fish in a medium-size saucepan and add the wine,
water, parsley, and thyme. Bring to a boil and reduce the
heat to a simmer. Cook for 10 minutes. The fish should be
hot and flaky; don't overcook it. Add the lemon juice.
Remove from heat.

Sauté the garlic in olive oil. Cook the pasta, drain it, and
pour it into a bowl. Pour in all of the fish and its cooking liquid plus the sautéed garlic. Toss. Serve while hot.

Makes four portions; 2 starch, 1 fat, and 4 protein per serving.

SALMON CROQUETTES

If you select canned salmon with the bones still in, you'll be
eating a superb calcium source. Many people object to the
texture of the bones. You can reduce this complaint by
mashing and chopping the salmon when the recipe calls for
mixing. Look for salmon labeled as "wild" instead of farm
raised. This recipe makes twelve croquettes. If you don't eat
them all at one meal, simply freeze them.

1 can salmon, drained   ½ cup finely chopped green
(14¾–ounce size)   pepper
1 cup dried bread crumbs   1 egg
¼ cup low-calorie mayonnaise   1 teaspoon prepared mustard
½ cup finely chopped onion   1 teaspoon Worcestershire sauce

Preheat the oven to 350°F. Mix all the ingredients, reserving
½ cup of bread crumbs. Mix until all the ingredients are
well blended. Shape into twelve cone-shaped croquettes.
Roll the croquettes in the remaining bread crumbs. Bake on
a slightly greased cookie sheet for 15 minutes. Serve topped
with Yogurt Dill Sauce.

Makes four three-croquette portions; 1 starch, 1 fat, and 4 protein per serving.

YOGURT DILL SAUCE: Mix 1 cup plain yogurt, 2 teaspoons dried dill or 1 tablespoon fresh minced dill, and 2 teaspoons lemon peel chopped fine or grated (buy a pesticide-free or unwaxed lemon).

Makes four ¼-cup servings; ¼ milk per serving.

ONE MORE FISH DISH

When I make this dish I like to buy a small portion of two or three different types of fish. For instance, I might have 5 ounces each of cod, haddock, and wild salmon. It's a great way to vary the recipe and to compare the flavors of the various fish.

1 pound fish (cod, haddock, wild salmon) or any combination that equals 1 pound
6 tablespoons olive oil

2 tablespoons fresh lemon juice
1 teaspoon Dijon mustard
1 tablespoon chopped fresh dill, parsley, or chives

Cut the fish into 2-inch cubes. Arrange on a 9-inch microwave-safe glass pie plate. Cover with a microwave-safe glass plate. Cook in the microwave on high power for 3 minutes.* Remove cover carefully; it will be hot. Rotate the fish so that any undercooked fish is moved to the outside of the dish. Cook 1 minute more, covered, on high power.

Mix the remaining ingredients together. Pour over the fish and let rest for 2 to 3 minutes to finish cooking. I like to serve this over hot pasta or cooked rice.

Makes four portions; 1 fat and 4 protein per serving.

---

*The cooking times are given for a 700-watt microwave with a carousel unit. Small ovens may require longer cooking times.

BROWN RICE AND BROCCOLI

I absolutely love brown rice cooked with wheat berries. It gives a gourmet touch without any fuss at all. My supermarket doesn't carry wheat berries, so I buy them in a specialty food shop or the health food store.

1 clove garlic, or 1 small onion, chopped	½ teaspoon salt (optional)
	3 cups broccoli, chopped
1 tablespoon olive oil	(1 large head)
1 cup brown rice	1 pound tofu, cubed
½ cup wheat berries	1 tablespoon soy sauce
3 cups boiling water	3 ounces cheddar cheese, grated

Sauté the garlic (or onion) in the oil in a heavy 10-inch skillet for 1 minute. Add the rice and wheat berries, cook 1 minute, and stir. Add the boiling water and salt. Bring to a boil, stir, and cook for 30 minutes, covered, on low heat.

Add the chopped broccoli and cook 5 minutes more, or until the broccoli is tender. If the rice looks dry, add another ¼ cup of water when the broccoli is added (you don't want the rice to dry out or it will burn). Toss in the tofu and soy sauce. Mix all the ingredients, sprinkle with grated cheese, and cover. Remove from heat and let rest for 2 to 3 minutes, or until cheese melts.

Makes three portions; 2 starch, 1 fat, 2 vegetable, and 3 protein per serving.

BEAUTIFUL BEAN AND VEGGIE SALAD

This is easy but very pretty and delicious. I developed it one day when I had to get something on the table fast and only had leftovers to work with. It was a hit!

1 can kidney beans, rinsed	1½ cups cooked chopped broccoli
10 black olives, sliced	
1½ cups cooked corkscrew noodles (rotini)	2 tablespoons low-calorie Italian dressing

Mix all ingredients together. Serve warm or refrigerate for 1 hour.

Makes three portions; 1 vegetable and 2 starch per serving.

CURRIED CHICKEN

This is a great way to use up leftover chicken or turkey. If you think you don't like curry, try this recipe, but put in only the amount of curry you think you can handle. If you refuse to eat curry, substitute an equal amount of dried dill.

1½ cups cubed, cooked chicken   *¾ cup plain yogurt*
(about 12 ounces)   *1 tablespoon curry powder*
1 tablespoon mayonnaise   *½ cup sliced red grapes*

Toss the cubed chicken with mayonnaise and yogurt. Sprinkle with curry; fold until well blended. Stir in the grapes. Serve on lettuce or in pita bread.

Makes three portions; ¼ milk, 1 fat, 1 fruit, and 3 protein per serving.

QUICK-COOKING CHILI

1 pound ground beef or ground   *1½ cups canned crushed*
turkey or textured vegetable   *tomatoes*
protein   *1 tablespoon chili powder,*
½ onion, chopped   *or ½ package of taco seasoning*
2 cups kidney beans   *mix*
(16-ounce can)   *salt (optional)*
2 cups corn (fresh or frozen)

Sauté the ground beef in a large saucepan on medium heat for 5 minutes. Drain off the fat. Add the onion, sauté 2 to 3 minutes more. Add the beans, corn, tomatoes, and the chili powder or taco seasoning. Simmer for 10 minutes. Taste and add more chili powder or salt if desired.

Makes five portions; 2 starch, 1 fat, 2 vegetable, and 3 protein per serving.

Textured Vegetable Protein—What Is It and Where Do I Get It?

Textured vegetable protein is a replacement for ground meat made mostly from soybeans. It might sound exotic, but I promise it is easy to use and you should give it a try at least once. I recommend it because it contains no saturated fat (the fat that clogs our arteries) and it is a good protein source. I buy it dry by the pound in my health food store—it looks like a cereal, but when added to recipes it absorbs the flavor and water and "bulks up." I also like frozen Morningstar Farms Veggie Crumbles, available in the freezer case. Follow the package instructions on portion to use to replace one pound of ground beef.

Food	Calories	Protein (g)	Total Fat (g)
3 ounces ground turkey cooked	193	22.4	2.8
3 ounces turkey sausage	135	12	7.9
3.5 ounces ground beef broiled	280	28.2	17.6
3 ounces pork sausage	300	15.9	25.2
Morningstar Farms Veggie Crumbles, ⅔ cup	80	10	2.5

BROCCOLI SALAD

Keep a batch of this in your refrigerator. It's a tasty, easy way to get healthy veggies.

1½ cups broccoli cut into
1-inch pieces
½ cup carrot chunks (cut carrot
in half lengthwise, then into
1-inch chunks)
2 tablespoons Italian dressing

Steam the vegetables for 5 minutes. Or sprinkle the vegetables with water and microwave covered in a microwave-safe dish for 3 minutes at full power, then stir and cook 1 minute more.

Put the cooked vegetables in a bowl and toss with the salad dressing. Serve warm or chilled.

Makes two 1-cup portions; 1 fat and 2 vegetable per serving. Use low-calorie dressing to reduce the fat by half.

QUICK SPAGHETTI SAUCE

Because of the added vegetables, this is more like a rata-touille than a conventional spaghetti sauce. Serve it over your favorite pasta.

1 pound ground beef or turkey or textured vegetable protein
2 cups tomato puree or crushed whole tomatoes
1 teaspoon oregano

1 cup any combination of chopped zucchini, mushrooms, and green peppers
1 tablespoon green capers (optional)
5–10 pitted Greek olives (optional)

Sauté the ground beef in a saucepan for 5 minutes on medium heat. Drain the fat and add the tomatoes, oregano, and vegetables. Bring to a boil, and then simmer on low for 2 minutes.

Makes four 1-cup portions; 1 vegetable and 4 protein per serving.

VEGETABLE MEAT LOAF

This is a great way to get some extra veggies. The vegeta-bles add flavor as well as nutrients to the meat loaf.

1 pound lean ground beef or ground turkey
2 cups finely grated vegetables, any combination: carrots, zucchini, mushrooms, green beans, green peppers, onion

1 cup crushed crackers, unsweetened flake cereal, or bread crumbs
salt and pepper
1 egg

Preheat the oven to 350°F. Mix all the ingredients in a bowl until they are all well blended. Press into an 8-inch by 4-inch loaf pan. Bake for 50 minutes or until done. After 20 minutes of cooking, pour off accumulated grease and continue cooking.

Makes four portions; 1 starch, 1 vegetable, and 4 protein per serving.

VEGETABLE STEW

Here's an easy recipe that can use any green you have available. Green leafy vegetables are a great way to get extra nutrition.

1 clove garlic, chopped
1 tablespoon olive oil
1 pound chopped greens
(spinach, kale, turnip greens,
or any combination)
4 cups chicken or vegetable
broth

¼ pound thin spaghetti broken
into 1-inch pieces
1 pound firm tofu cut into
1-inch cubes (optional)

Gently cook the garlic in the oil over low heat until tender. Do not brown. Add the well-washed chopped greens and mix. Cover and cook over low heat for 5 minutes. Add the broth, bring to a boil, and add the pieces of raw pasta. Reduce heat to low, cover, and simmer for 20 minutes. If you're adding tofu, stir it in after 15 minutes of cooking and let it simmer with the vegetables for the remaining 5 minutes.

Serve in bowls with good crusty bread, some grated cheese, and even a splash of soy sauce.

Makes four good-size portions; 1 starch, 1 fat, and 1 vegetable per serving. If you add the tofu, count it as 1 protein per serving.

HUNTER'S PIE

This is a variation of shepherd's pie, only easier because you don't need to mash the potatoes. I also use either fresh or frozen peas and corn, depending on what's available. They will cook or thaw once in the oven.

1 pound ground beef or ground
turkey or textured vegetable
protein
2 tablespoons chili sauce
1 cup peas, fresh or frozen

1 cup corn, fresh or frozen
4 small potatoes, sliced thin
4 teaspoons margarine, melted
salt and pepper (optional)

Preheat the oven to 350°F. Lightly oil a microwave- and oven-safe 1-quart casserole dish. Cook the ground beef for 3 minutes on high power in the microwave. Drain the fat, mash the lumps, and mix in the chili sauce. Some of the meat will still be red. Layer the peas and corn over the meat, then arrange the sliced potatoes in a circular pattern on top of the vegetables. Drizzle the margarine on top of the potatoes, sprinkle with salt and pepper if desired, and bake for 40 minutes, until the potatoes are tender.

Makes four portions; 2 starch, 1 fat, and 4 protein per serving.

Whole Grains

Whole grains include whole wheat, whole rye, whole corn, whole barley, and popcorn. Any items made from these ingredients are nutrition stars. They are credited with preventing heart disease, controlling weight, and managing diabetes. The 2005 U.S. Dietary Guidelines recommend that women eat at least 3 servings of whole grains daily, men 3 to 4 servings, and children 1½ to 3 servings daily. A serving is defined as an 80-calorie portion or 1 slice of bread, ½ cup cooked pasta or rice, or 1 cup of cereal. When a breastfeeding mother starts the day with a whole grain cereal (1 serving) and includes two slices of whole wheat bread (2 servings) at lunch, she's got what she needs; any extra servings are a bonus.

Whole Grain Cooking Primer

Don't be intimidated by these unfamiliar grains. You cook them almost exactly the same way you would prepare white or brown rice. Use water or broth, season with salt, and add a little oil.

Barley Use in soup or serve as a side dish like rice. Kids love it when it is thoroughly cooked, soft, and creamy.

Combine ½ cup barley in 2½ cups water or broth. Bring to a boil, stir, cover, and simmer 45 minutes.

Bulgur (Kasha) Good in soups and chili.

Combine 1 cup of bulgur with 2 cups water. Add salt to taste and 1 teaspoon oil. Bring to a boil, stir, cover, reduce heat and cook 20 minutes until tender.

Couscous Small grains that cook quickly.

Bring 2 cups of water to a boil. Stir in ¾ cup couscous. Remove from heat. Cover and let stand for 5 minutes, or until the liquid is absorbed.

Quinoa A nutty-tasting grain.

Bring 2 cups of water or broth to a boil. Stir in 1 cup quinoa and 1 teaspoon canola oil. Cover, reduce heat, and cook for 20 minutes or until tender.

Try the Brown Rice and Broccoli recipe on page 188 for another delicious whole grain recipe.

Meals in a Blender

Busy new mothers may find it helpful to keep ready-to-drink nutritious shakes on hand in the refrigerator. When I was home with Sarah and too busy to make a snack, I relied on these. I made a batch in the morning and sipped it throughout the day. It was something I could easily handle while I nursed my new daughter.

BANANA FRAPPÉ

1 cup low-fat milk   *1 ripe banana*
½ cup orange juice

Mix all ingredients in a blender. Serve in a tall glass or over ice.

Makes two large portions; ½ milk and 1 fruit per serving.

ORANGE CREAM

Some mothers just don't like plain milk. Here's a fabulous recipe that contains over 250 milligrams of calcium in one serving.

1 6-ounce can frozen orange   *1 teaspoon vanilla extract*
juice   *1 cup water*
1 cup nonfat dry milk   *2½ cups ice cubes*

Blend all ingredients in the blender, adding ice cubes gradually.

Makes three portions; 1 milk and 2 fruit per serving.

Crock-Pot Cooking

Crock-Pot cooking is ideal for busy new moms. You can put the ingredients in the pot in the morning, and they will cook while you are out doing errands. Even if you stay at home for the day, you will have a meal that requires no tending to. To keep meals healthy, trim all visible fat from meats and remove skin from poultry. I always add a generous portion of vegetables to my meals.

CHICKEN CACCIATORE

I love this dish because it is so flavorful. All I have to do is serve it with a side of pasta and I have a complete meal. The recipe contains a lot of vegetables and it's a good protein source, too. I keep the chopped vegetables about one inch in size—any smaller and they can get lost, though the flavor and nutrition remain.

4 chicken thighs, bone and skin removed
1 green pepper, chopped
1 yellow squash, chopped
1 zucchini, chopped

8 ounces mushrooms, sliced
1 28-ounce can chopped tomatoes
1 bay leaf

Place the chicken in the bottom of a Crock-Pot and add all ingredients on top. Cover and cook on low setting for 8 to 10 hours or on high for 4 hours.

Makes 4 portions; 2 vegetable and 2 protein.

CLASSIC POT ROAST

Let this cook all day until the meat is tender. Remove the meat and vegetables and add a slurry of water and cornstarch to thicken the juices into a gravy.

4 potatoes, peeled and cubed
1 beef bouillon cube
1 16-ounce bag baby carrots
1 onion, peeled and quartered

1 pound frozen green beans
3–4 pound pot roast
Water to cover the ingredients halfway, about 2 cups

Place the potatoes in the pot, along with the bouillon cube, and top with the vegetables. Center the pot roast on top and add the water. Cover and cook on low for 8 to 10 hours.

This can be used to make several meals; 4 protein, 2 vegetable, and 1 starch per serving.

Healthy Desserts

Desserts can be a part of our meals if we choose those that provide nutrition as well as taste. The choices that follow are low in fat but high in flavor and nutrition.

YOGURT SUNDAE

This isn't exotic, but it looks pretty enough to be a fattening, forbidden food. I make it in a champagne goblet for an elegant presentation.

1 cup yogurt (plain or vanilla)
¼ cup granola or other crunchy cereal
½ cup fruit, any type

Put ½ cup yogurt in the bottom of the dish and top with the granola. Layer the remaining yogurt on top with the fresh fruit.

Makes one portion; 1 starch, 1 milk, and 1 fruit per serving.

CHOCOLATE CREAM

One of my patients gave me this recipe. It is a delicious no-cook pudding, rich in calcium and protein.

12 ounces extra-firm silk tofu   *1 tablespoon Splenda or ¼ cup*
1 tablespoon vanilla   *sugar*
                                                   4 tablespoons cocoa powder

Put all ingredients in a food processor or blender. Puree until smooth. Serve garnished with fresh fruit.

Makes two portions; ½ milk per serving.

WHOLE WHEAT BREAD PUDDING

Here is a way to get fiber, calcium, zinc, and protein all in one dish. What a great way to get nutrition!

2 slices whole wheat bread,   *2 tablespoons honey, or*
toasted   *1 tablespoon honey and*
1 cup milk   *1 tablespoon molasses or*
1 egg, slightly beaten   *maple syrup*

Preheat the oven to 350°F. Tear the toast into 1-inch pieces. Mix all the ingredients in a bowl until the bread is well coated.

Pour into a lightly greased 4-cup baking dish. Bake for 30 minutes. Serve topped with ½ cup ice milk.

Makes two portions; 1 starch, ¼ milk, 1 daily option, and ½ protein exchange per serving.

INDIAN PUDDING

This is one of my absolute all-time favorites and very easy to make.

1 cup cornmeal   3 tablespoons molasses
2 cups 1 percent milk

Mix all ingredients in a microwave-safe glass dish. Cook in the microwave for 3 minutes on high power, uncovered. Stir. Cook for 2 more minutes. Let rest, covered, for 2 minutes. The pudding should be thick and creamy. If it gets too thick, stir in ¼ to ½ cup more milk.

Makes four portions; 1 starch, ½ milk, and 1 daily option exchange per serving.

BAKED PEARS

These can be prepared in the microwave or in a conventional oven. Topped with yogurt and served with a crisp gingersnap, they are refreshing and wholesome.

1 pear   1 tablespoon brown sugar
½ cup boiling water

Slice the pear in half and remove the core and stem. Place the cut side down on a lightly oiled baking dish. Mix together the sugar and water and pour over pear halves.

   Microwave oven: Cook on high power, uncovered, for 3 minutes. Cover and let rest for 2 minutes.

   Conventional oven: Bake at 350°F, covered, for 20 minutes.

Makes one portion; 1 fruit and 1 daily option per serving.

BLUEBERRY SAUCE

We try to keep the intake of simple sugars low in our house. To use less syrup on pancakes and waffles, we came up with this fabulous creation. When the blueberries cook they release their own juices, making "syrup."

1 cup fresh or frozen blueberries   2 tablespoons maple syrup

Combine the fruit and syrup in a small saucepan. Cook for 10 minutes on medium heat, covered. Allow to cool. Use as you would maple syrup.

Makes one portion; 1 fruit and 1 daily option per serving.

FAT-FREE CHOCOLATE SAUCE

I love the taste of chocolate. Cocoa powder by itself is almost fat free. This recipe has no added fat and it satisfies my craving for chocolate. Use it to top ice milk or frozen yogurt.

2 tablespoons unsweetened cocoa
1 to 2 tablespoons sugar
2 tablespoons water (instead of water you can try a sweet liqueur like Grand Marnier and omit half the sugar)

Mix the sugar and cocoa in a small, heavy saucepan. Add the liquid and stir over medium-low heat. The powder will eventually absorb the liquid. Heat until the mixture is well combined and some of the liquid evaporates, about 2 minutes. Remove from heat before boiling or it will become too thick.

Makes two portions; 1 daily option per serving. The sugar and cocoa have no redeeming nutritional qualities, so they can't be counted in any of the food groups. Use this just occasionally.

GOOD QUICK CAKE

Here's a simple, tender cake that can be prepared and on the table within 30 minutes. Read the variations below to discover ways to dress it up by adding some special mix-ins. Another super plus is that there is no added fat in this cake—the only fat comes from the eggs.

1½ cups all-purpose flour	¼ teaspoon salt
⅔ cup sugar	1 cup yogurt, plain
2 teaspoons baking powder	2 eggs
½ teaspoon baking soda	

Preheat the oven to 375°F. Mix all the dry ingredients together. In a separate bowl, combine the yogurt and eggs. Mix thoroughly. Fold the yogurt mixture into the dry ingredients until blended, but do not overmix. Pour into a lightly oiled tube-cake pan or an 8-inch square cake pan. Bake for 20 minutes or until the top is golden.

Makes twelve portions; 1 starch per serving.

BLUEBERRY CAKE: Gently fold in ¾ cup fresh or frozen blueberries after all of the ingredients have been mixed. Bake as directed.

BANANA CAKE: Mix 2 small, very ripe bananas (approximately ½ cup) into the yogurt and egg mixture. Mash it in well, fold the yogurt mixture into the dry ingredients, and bake as directed.

Something to Snack On
There are no bad snacks—just bad snack choices! Choose foods that are nutritious and you actually help your body.

Munchies

These are good snacks to keep around for when you've got to have something to eat but don't want to eat high-fat, not-so-good-for-you junk food. In chapter 12 read about the everyday snacks I suggest once you stop breastfeeding.

- Air-popped popcorn
- Angel food cake (serve with fruit and low-fat yogurt or ice milk)

- Graham crackers
- Animal crackers
- Hard candy (Fat-free candy and gumdrops can help those of you with an urge for sugar. They contain no vitamins or minerals. If they prevent a binge on candy bars, then they can be considered a good snack choice.)
- Gumdrops
- Fruit
- Sliced peppers
- Pretzels
- Rice cakes
- Breadsticks
- Water ice/Popsicles/fruit pops

Stamina Snacks

These snacks have protein to carry you to the next meal.

- Hard-cooked eggs
- Cheese melted on a soft tortilla
- Low-fat cottage cheese on a cracker
- Peanut butter on graham crackers or rice cakes
- Nuts (careful how many you eat—high in fat)
- Soup—choose a broth soup with meat or beans
- Yogurt
- Mini pizza—melted cheese on an English muffin topped with tomato and oregano
- Hummus with pita bread
- Baked potato with a slice of cheese melted on top

BE A SMART SHOPPER

There are a lot of foods at the supermarket or health food store that are easy to prepare and good for you, too. The lists below give my recommendations for nutritious, low-fat foods. In most cases, the simpler the food, the more nutritious it is. A fresh broccoli stalk is a better nutrition buy than a package of frozen chopped broccoli with cheese sauce.

The emphasis in my selections is to keep fat intake low. This doesn't mean that breastfeeding mothers have unique fat requirements. All of us—new mothers, grandparents, fathers, brothers, and sisters—should be more careful about the amount of fat we put into our bodies.

Reading Labels

Food packages list ingredients with the predominant item first. A sweetened cereal with sugar listed as a first ingredient would be loaded with sugar. A cereal with sugar as the third or fourth ingredient would have a much lower sugar content. Be leery of labels that tout "No Cholesterol" or "99% Fat Free," as these claims can be misleading. For instance, several brands of peanut butter claim that they have no cholesterol. The consumer would assume that these are better products than the ones that do not carry the no-cholesterol claims. The truth is that no peanut butter contains cholesterol because peanuts are plant foods, and only animal foods contain cholesterol. Words like *fresh* and *all natural* don't carry much meaning, either. Your best bet is to read labels carefully and try to choose as many wholesome, unprocessed foods as possible.

Four areas to pay attention to when reading labels

- **Servings:** When using a food label, start by determining the true serving you will actually eat. The package label on page 203 describes a one-cup portion, but if you eat the two portions the box actually contains, double everything.
- **Fat:** The saturated fat content and *trans*-fat content are more important than the total fat because if these are low, the remaining fats are the ones good for our heart.

Sample Label for
Macaroni & Cheese

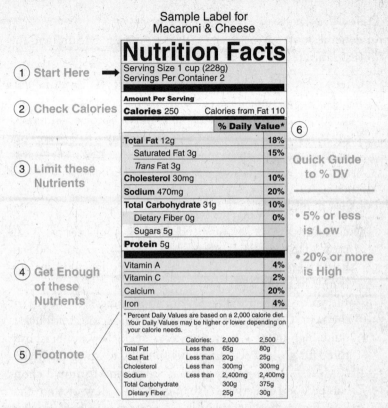

① Start Here ➡

② Check Calories

③ Limit these
Nutrients

④ Get Enough
of these
Nutrients

⑤ Footnote

Nutrition Facts

Serving Size 1 cup (228g)
Servings Per Container 2

Amount Per Serving

Calories 250   Calories from Fat 110

	% Daily Value*	⑥
Total Fat 12g	18%	
Saturated Fat 3g	15%	
Trans Fat 3g		
Cholesterol 30mg	10%	
Sodium 470mg	20%	
Total Carbohydrate 31g	10%	
Dietary Fiber 0g	0%	
Sugars 5g		
Protein 5g		
Vitamin A	4%	
Vitamin C	2%	
Calcium	20%	
Iron	4%	

* Percent Daily Values are based on a 2,000 calorie diet.
Your Daily Values may be higher or lower depending on
your calorie needs.

	Calories:	2,000	2,500
Total Fat	Less than	65g	80g
Sat Fat	Less than	20g	25g
Cholesterol	Less than	300mg	300mg
Sodium	Less than	2,400mg	2,400mg
Total Carbohydrate		300g	375g
Dietary Fiber		25g	30g

Quick Guide
to % DV

_____

• 5% or less
is Low

• 20% or more
is High

Source: Center for Food Safety and Applied Nutrition, USDA.

- **Sugar:** Sugar content is only useful when comparing similar products. For example, if you compare the sugar content between brands of peanut butter, you are using it correctly. If you compare the sugar content in yogurt to the sugar content in cheese and conclude that cheese is a better snack choice because it carries no sugar, you would be incorrect. The sugar in yogurt is naturally occurring, not an added sugar.

- **Calcium:** Use the calcium percentage to choose foods rich in calcium. Thirty percent calcium means that the portion of food carries 300 milligrams of calcium, the amount in one cup of milk.

Dairy Products
In general, look for the foods with the greatest calcium and the lowest saturated and *trans*-fat content.

Cheese: Try the low-fat varieties, including the lower-fat cottage cheeses and "diet" slices of American cheese.
Milk: Low-fat milk of all kinds, buttermilk, chocolate skim milk.
Yogurt: Try yogurt with a fat content of only 0 to 3 grams per eight-ounce serving.

Meats
Look for items low in saturated fat and rich in protein.

Deli Counter: Chicken or sliced turkey is your best bet. Lean meats like roast beef, turkey ham, turkey pastrami, and lean ham are okay choices. Try to skip the high-fat cold cuts, pastrami, and hot dogs.
Poultry: All chicken and turkey are good choices; try not to eat the skin. Cornish hens are a good choice, too, but duck is quite high in fat. Ground turkey and chicken can be substituted for ground beef in recipes, helping to lower fat intake.
Red Meat: All lean meats such as steaks and trimmed chops can be good selections. When cooking a stew or soup that calls for ground beef, buy lean or extra-lean beef for that recipe because the fat will be cooked in. The less expensive, higher-fat ground beef can be used if the fat can be drained off during cooking. Avoid high-fat meats such as bacon, sausage, short ribs, corned beef, and pastrami. If you do have these meats, keep the portions small.
Fish: All plain, unprocessed fish is a good choice. Don't be afraid to use frozen fish. It's tasty when baked and usually costs less than fresh fish.

Fats
Compare saturated and *trans*-fat content. Choose products with the lowest content of both.

Oils: All vegetable oils are cholesterol free because they are extracted from vegetables. Vegetables carry fats that are thought to be good for us; these are known as polyunsaturated and monounsaturated fats. Oils vary in their content of polyunsaturated and monounsaturated fats, flavor, and cooking properties. Good choices include canola, olive, safflower, soybean, sunflower, corn, peanut, and sesame oils. Butter and margarine both contain an equal number of calories. Butter contains cholesterol and saturated fats that can raise a person's blood cholesterol. Margarine, however, contains no cholesterol and very small amounts of saturated fat. As of 2006 all margarine products will list the *trans*-fat content, making it easy to choose those without *trans*-fat. Lard also contains saturated fat, and shortenings are treated in such a way that much of the fat they contain is also saturated. Remember, all oils contain approximately 45 calories per teaspoon.

Salad Dressing and Mayonnaise: Read labels and select one that supplies less than 5 grams of fat per serving. Those made with olive or canola oil are my favorite choices.

Fruit

Use labels to choose items low in sugar and rich in fiber. All fresh fruits are good choices. I often treat myself to the more expensive "exotic" fruits like papaya or mango—they seem like more special desserts. Frozen fruits and canned fruit prepared without sugar are good choices, too. Be cautious of dried fruits. They're easy to snack on but carry a lot of calories.

Vegetables

All fresh veggies are great. In fact, I think they make a good quick snack: a half cup of any vegetable can be chopped and ready to eat after just two minutes of cooking in the microwave. Canned vegetables always contain more salt than fresh varieties unless they are specially marked. Plain frozen vegetables are great, too.

Watch out for the vegetables that are frozen with butter or cheese sauces; they're packed with fat calories.

Starches

Bread: Most breads are naturally low in fat and are packed with B vitamins and healthy carbohydrates. Exceptions are cheese breads, butter breads, and rolls. Baked goods such as croissants, muffins, and biscuits are higher in fat than sliced breads. Try to get into the habit of buying whole grain breads. They contain more fiber than white bread and therefore can be a better health choice.

Cereals: These grain foods are a terrific way to get nutrition. When selecting cereal, try to buy the whole grain types without added sugar or fat (granola cereals can be quite high in fat). Read labels and buy a cereal that contains 0 to 3 grams of fat per serving and 2 grams or more of fiber.

Pasta and Rice: These are superb foods when purchased in their simple, unadorned state. Ready-to-serve brown rice is worth the extra money for the time it can save. Convenience pasta and rice packages that require lots of added butter or margarine are not good choices. When I prepare these items I reduce the amount of fat or oil suggested by one-half or two-thirds. The ramen-style noodles are very high in fat because they are fried after cooking, then dried and packaged.

Frozen Foods

If you shop smart, you can find some healthy foods in the freezer case. Most are ready to serve, which makes them very useful to new mothers. Your best choices are simple foods like the frozen fruits and vegetables. Keep bags of frozen vegetable combinations on hand for quick meals. Frozen rice or pasta dishes without sauces are good, too (we love the ready-to-cook frozen raviolis, pierogis, and manicottis). Frozen pizza crust lets you make your own healthy pizza in just minutes. Sprinkle a frozen crust with low-fat cheese, a bit of pureed tomato sauce, and fresh or frozen vegetables and cook at 350°F until the cheese melts and the veggies are tender—about ten to fifteen minutes.

Frozen Desserts: Fruit bars, frozen low-fat yogurt, Italian ices, and fudge bars are good selections. Ice milk is good, too. Premium ice creams contain much more fat and should be saved for special treats. *Generally, the more expensive the ice cream, the higher its fat content.* Frozen frosted cakes and pies aren't great choices, but frozen plain cakes can be.

Frozen Entrees: More and more frozen dinners are being slimmed down by their manufacturers, and these can be good quick choices for hurried moms. They all contain more sodium than the same food prepared from scratch. In many cases, the low-calorie frozen dinners may be too low in calories for you. Most supply only 250 to 350 calories; a breastfeeding mother will need closer to 600 calories at a meal. To add the extra low-fat calories you'll need, try eating a couple of slices of whole wheat bread with just a bit of butter or margarine spread on or a yogurt, milk, or even extra vegetables.

Frozen burritos are quick meals if you like and can tolerate beans. They contain about 350 calories each, with 30 percent of those calories coming from fat.

Canned Foods

All canned meats, mixed dishes, and vegetables have added salt unless they are specifically marked "no salt added." The only exception to this is canned fruit, which can have added sugar. Use the sugar and fiber content listed on canned fruit labels to choose the best products. I always keep a supply of broth-based canned soups on hand. I know they have more sodium than the ones I make from scratch, but let's face it—I can't always make my own broth. I prefer the broth soups over cream soups because the latter have more fat. I also like canned beans because they are more convenient than soaking and cooking my own. I just rinse the salt off before using. I rarely if ever buy canned mixed dinners because I don't like the taste. However, a canned chili or stew might appeal to you, though it will be higher in sodium and probably lower in protein and vegetables than one you make yourself.

Seasonings

All seasonings, including herbs and spices, are okay to use. Herbs and spices with salt added are best avoided; I recommend unsalted varieties, for example, onion powder over onion salt. Check out your local health food store. Most sell herbs and seasonings in bulk at a fraction of the price sold in supermarkets. Breastfeeding mothers who feel that some seasonings bother their babies can simply avoid or reduce these seasonings while nursing.

GRANDMA'S BEST BETS

My mother is a superb cook, and she graciously volunteered to stay for a week when Sarah was born, to help out her overwhelmed daughter. Not only did she do a magnificent job caring for me, David, and the house; she also left me with a freezer full of delicious meals. She left a sliced, cooked pot roast, a batch of great tomato sauce in two-cup portions, and the following recipes, ready to reheat. If your mother comes to visit, ask her to put a few of these in the freezer, too.

CHICKEN IN THE POT

This is a recipe my mother gave me for quick cooking. It never made its way into the freezer—we ate it too fast.

2 cloves garlic   *4 cups water*
1 3-pound whole chicken   *1 onion, peeled*

½ teaspoon thyme	4 carrots, peeled and cut in chunks
3 sprigs parsley	4 stalks celery, chopped
6 peppercorns	4 potatoes, peeled and cut in
1 bay leaf	quarters

Place a clove of garlic in each end of the chicken. Put chicken in a heavy pot along with neck and gizzards and remaining ingredients. Bring to a boil, cover, and simmer for 1 hour. Serve the chicken on a platter surrounded by the cooked vegetables. Use the stock as a gravy for the potatoes.

Makes about 8 portions; 1 starch, 1 vegetable, and 4 protein per serving.

HAMBURGER SOUP

This makes a good-size pot; you can eat some and then freeze the rest. It contains protein, vegetables, and starch in one meal. Accompany the soup with a glass of milk and some sliced bread or a salad and you have a healthy, tasty meal. If you allow this to cool in the refrigerator before eating, all the fat rises to the top and can be skimmed off. This trick saves lots of fat calories without harming the taste at all.

2 onions, chopped	1 bay leaf
1 tablespoon margarine or	9 peppercorns
vegetable oil	½ teaspoon thyme
½ to 1 pound lean ground beef,	3 ribs celery, chopped
turkey, or textured soy protein	3 carrots, sliced
2 cans consommé, or 4 cups	2 potatoes, diced
broth	3 tablespoons fresh parsley,
1 28-ounce can whole tomatoes	chopped

Sauté the onions in the margarine or vegetable oil until tender. Add the ground meat and cook 5 minutes. Drain the fat. Add the consommé plus 3 cans of water or broth. Omit water if using broth. Stir in tomatoes, bay leaf, peppercorns, thyme, chopped celery, sliced carrots, diced potatoes, and parsley. Bring to a boil; quickly reduce to low heat, and simmer for at least 1 hour. Best if made early in the day.

Makes four portions; 1 starch, 1 fat, 2 vegetable, and 2 to 4 protein per serving.

CHILIBURGER SOUP

You can use ground beef, ground turkey, or textured vegetable protein in this recipe. This soup contains protein, vegetables, and starch from the barley.

2 onions, chopped	1 32-ounce can tomato juice
1 tablespoon vegetable oil	½ teaspoon to 1 tablespoon chili
3 celery stalks, chopped	powder
1 pound ground meat	½ cup pearl barley, uncooked

Sauté the onions in the oil until tender. Add the celery and ground meat and cook for 5 minutes, mashing any lumps. Drain the fat. Add the tomato juice, chili powder, and barley. Bring to a boil, then reduce heat and simmer for 1 hour.

Makes four portions; 1 fat, 2 vegetable, and 4 protein per serving.

VARIATION: In the last 10 minutes of cooking, add 1 cup of any fresh vegetable, such as corn, peas, green beans, or zucchini. If using frozen vegetables, add in the last 5 minutes of cooking. This will add half of a vegetable exchange.

WHEN FRIENDS ASK, "WHAT CAN I DO?"—TELL THEM!

I received many wonderful gifts from friends and family, but one of the most memorable and timely was from my neighbor Valerie. Sarah wasn't even a week old and it was early afternoon.

I heard a knock on my door and opened it to find Valerie standing there with a bag full of food. She had a large salad, a fresh vegetable quiche, a full bottle of wine, and an entire chocolate cake from the bakery. David and I were absolutely thrilled to have a complete meal delivered to the house. We savored every bit and drank small celebratory glasses of wine. I must confess that the chocolate cake went quite quickly.

So when friends ask what they can do, take them up on their generosity and give them some ideas.

- Ask them to make you some home-cooked food like a stew or casserole.
- If you don't feel comfortable with that, ask them to go to the store and buy you some nutritious, ready-to-eat foods. A quick trip to the supermarket can yield a fresh roasted chicken, a large salad from the salad bar, and a loaf of bread.
- If you have older children, ask friends if they could take the kids for a while so you can have some time alone with the new baby.
- If they are really good friends, let them do the laundry or clean the house.
- If they want to help you out with a gift, suggest a certificate for a cleaning service or a diaper service.
- If you need a breast pump when you return to work, maybe they would want to help you out with the cost of renting one.
- My good friend Marilyn gave me a card with a coupon in it to be redeemed for five hours of babysitting. I didn't use this until Sarah was about four months old, but it was a wonderful gift and it gave me a sense of independence, knowing that I could count on one of my best friends to take care of Sarah when I needed time to myself.

11
QUESTIONS, ANSWERS, AND PROBLEM SOLVING

SOME COMMON CONCERNS

When I first became a mother I kept a daily diary. Most of these questions are taken from the problems and concerns that I wrote down. I think many new mothers also face these issues, so this question-and-answer section was added to help find answers to these common concerns.

How often should I let my baby nurse?

Breastfed babies do best if they can feed on demand. In the beginning, this helps to establish a good milk supply. It takes about 1½ hours for breast milk to empty out of a baby's stomach. Your baby will probably want to feed every two to three hours, but some may want to eat every hour at the beginning. Breastfed babies often seem to eat more frequently than bottle-fed babies; there is nothing unusual about this.

How will I know if my baby is getting enough to eat?

Your baby should wet at least five to eight diapers every day. In the first months, he should have two to five bowel movements daily (this drops off after the second month). When you bring him for his first weight check at two weeks, he should be gaining weight and growing in length and head circumference. If he also appears happy and content, you can be pretty sure he's getting enough food.

I want to use a breast pump but I can't seem to get the hang of it. What should I do?

The letdown reflex is a complex but natural chain of events. When your baby suckles at your breast, hormones and chemicals in your body are triggered to send milk to your breast and baby. You need to establish the letdown reflex in order to pump successfully. This means relaxing. Find yourself a quiet spot and think about your baby. You can also try applying a warm facecloth to your breasts or giving yourself a gentle breast massage. Then place the pump over the areola and operate according to its instructions. Many mothers have reported better luck with electric pumps rather than with battery-powered or manual pumps. If this still doesn't work, hunt out a fellow mom who has successfully pumped, or contact the La Leche League or a lactation consultant for support. Most mothers find that with practice, pumping becomes easier.

All parts of the breast pump that come in contact with breast milk should be sterilizable or disposable. Keep this in mind when choosing a machine. Cleanliness and good hygiene will prevent infection.

What is a lactation consultant and how do I find one?

A lactation consultant is an allied health care worker with special training in assisting mothers with unusual and routine breastfeeding situations. Such a consultant provides education and is usually affiliated with a medical team. The International Board of Lactation Consultant Examiners (IBLCE) in Falls Church, Virginia, credentials individuals who want to offer professional breastfeeding counseling. To find a lactation consultant, ask your doctor or midwife, or look in the Resources section at the back of this book. The mothers I have talked with who needed and used a lactation consultant consider them lifesavers. One mother with a premature child said that if it were not for her lactation consultant, she never would have had enough support to nurse her baby boy. Another mother whose baby girl didn't nurse well was referred to a lactation consultant who arranged for the mother to try a special feeding device known as a Lact-Aid Nursing Trainer. The device worked wonders, and mother and baby had a healthy, happy nursing experience.

How can I find a qualified nutritionist?

Ask your health care provider for the name of a dietitian or nutritionist. If he or she can't recommend one, then look in the yellow pages. It doesn't really matter if they call themselves nutritionists or dietitians because the word *nutritionist* has no legal definition. Anyone from a vitamin salesman to a doctor can use the term. Do look for a registered dietitian (R.D.). These professionals have attended college and have completed advance studies in nutrition, either as interns or in a master's program in nutrition or a related field. They have also passed an extensive exam in nutrition, and they must keep up their registration by completing continuing education courses in nutrition every year. Many, but not all, states license dietitians. Licensed dietitians will use R.D. and L.D. (licensed dietitian) after their name.

To find a dietitian in your area go to www.eatright.org and click "find a dietitian."

What should I look for in a nursing bra?

A breastfeeding woman doesn't need to wear a bra if she doesn't want to, but a good nursing bra can give one's breasts extra support. For women who wear bras, it can make feeding time easier and more comfortable because the bra flap lifts easily, allowing the baby to feed. Select a bra that's all cotton because cotton breathes better than synthetics and allows extra moisture to evaporate, keeping you more comfortable. Avoid underwire-type nursing bras because the wires can block milk ducts and cause discomfort. Most women find that while nursing they need a bra that is one to two sizes larger than their prepregnancy bra.

What can I do if my breasts become engorged?

Breast engorgement isn't uncommon and it can be very uncomfortable. To relieve the discomfort, try warm heat such as a hot shower or moist cloth.

If your breast engorges, massage it before feeding the baby; you may also need to manually express some milk to soften the breast so your baby can latch on easier. Allow your baby to nurse at the engorged breast first—this is when he is most hungry and his sucking will help relieve engorgement.

The key to overcoming engorgement is to try to avoid it in the first place; feed early and frequently from birth on.

How can I prevent sore nipples?

Proper positioning of the baby at the breast can help, as can allowing your breast to air dry after each feeding. Of course this is a bit tough in public. When you're not at home, try wiping off any excess milk with a clean cloth moistened with plain water.

I'm a thirty-five-year-old mom. Does age affect how much milk I make?

A study of 155 mothers ranging in age from fifteen to thirty-seven years old was conducted and reported in *Human Lactation 2* (Plenum Press, 1986). The researchers studied how much milk these mothers made and its nutritional composition. Milk volume was not related to age. There were some differences in milk fat and lactose content between moms of different ages, but the significance of these findings is unclear. In short, older mothers (and there are many more of us these days) can breastfeed successfully.

If breast milk is the perfect food for baby, why is my pediatrician telling me to give him vitamins?

Breast milk is the perfect food for your baby because it is intensely rich in nutrients. Usually supplements are advised for vitamin D, vitamin K, and iron for the following reasons:

- **Vitamin D:** Recognizing that sunlight exposure, as a source of vitamin D, is difficult to determine, starting at two months of age the AAP and the CDC recommend 200 IU of vitamin D for all breastfed infants.
- **Vitamin K:** All babies are given a dose of vitamin K at birth to protect them against hemorrhaging. Regardless of the type of feeding method chosen for the baby, vitamin K injections are given as a safety measure.
- **Iron:** By the time a child is six months old, he needs to start eating foods rich in iron. If intakes of these foods are low, iron supplements will be recommended.

Most pediatricians do not recommend multivitamins for nursing babies because your breast milk supplies all the calories and nutrients needed (except for the occasional exceptions mentioned above). Mothers who eat absolutely no animal-based foods, including eggs, milk, and cheese, will need to take a B_{12} supplement so their breast milk is adequate in B_{12}. The DRI while breastfeeding is 2.8 micrograms per day.

My baby is now two months old and I want to lose weight. Can I try Weight Watchers or a liquid diet?

Liquid diets are not recommended for breastfeeding mothers. These regimens usually advise the dieter to take one diet drink at breakfast and one at lunch, and then eat a small meal at suppertime. Each diet drink provides only 250 to 300 calories. If supper weighs in at 500 calories, a mother following this diet would be eating less than 1,200 calories a day. At this level, she won't be able to meet her requirement for most nutrients, and her milk production may actually decline. So please, no liquid diets designed for rapid weight loss.

Weight Watchers has a menu designed for both pregnant women and nursing mothers. The group leaders of a Weight Watchers program might not be familiar with the recommended safe weight loss for nursing mothers or their unique nutritional needs. If you decide to use the Weight Watchers program, you must assume personal responsibility for getting enough food and losing weight slowly and safely.

Is it safe to take diet pills sold without a prescription?

No. Drugstore diet pills contain high levels of caffeine (as much as 200 to 280 milligrams in a day's dose). This is equivalent to drinking two to three extra cups of coffee per day. If these pills are consumed regularly, enough caffeine could accumulate in your breast milk to be harmful to your baby.

I'm worried about my baby's weight gain.

Rate of weight gain is an important indicator of health, but it's not the only factor, and slow weight gain alone doesn't mean a child is failing to thrive. Dr. Ruth Lawrence in *Breastfeeding: A Guide for the Medical Profession* suggests that a child who is slow to gain weight but "alert, bright and responsive" and developing appropriately should be classified as a slow gainer. A child who is not gaining weight, is apathetic, has a weak cry and poor skin tone, wets very few diapers, and passes few stools may be a true case of failure to thrive. Dr. Lawrence's book would be a good book to recommend to any physician needing more information on the development of the breastfeeding baby. While slow weight gain alone doesn't necessitate the use of supplemental formula, if your baby has any of the symptoms of failure to thrive, you need to work with your doctor to meet your baby's nutritional needs.

WEIGHT LOSS STRATEGIES AND BEHAVIOR MODIFICATION

Knowing what is good and healthy to eat is not all we need to help us eat better or lose weight. The way our families react to diet changes or altered exercise programs can make a big difference in our success in meeting our goals. If you feel you have problems that interfere with your ambitions for changing eating habits, you aren't alone. Most of us find that lack of time, our families' eating preferences, and the foods that friends drop off as gifts get in the way of our intended goals. And old eating habits die hard. The problems that follow may sound familiar to you. You'll be interested to see how you can turn them around to your advantage.

My husband works late, so I feed the children at five o'clock and eat with them. Even though I have already eaten, I'm hungry again when my husband gets home, and I pick enough to make up another meal. How can I stop eating the equivalent of two meals each night?

Eat your full meal at five o'clock and eat a planned snack later. A salad or some cooked vegetables or an appropriate snack such as a yogurt sundae could be enjoyed with your husband.

When friends drop by, they either bring something to munch on or I pull something out of the freezer. Most of the time I end up overeating. What can I do?

Talk with your friends. Tell them that you want to eat more healthily and ask them to help you out. Foods such as fruits and vegetables would be appropriate munchies. A tray of sliced fresh fruits sprinkled with lemon can be terrific. Or serve simple low-fat crackers, breadsticks, or pretzels with some really good tangy mustard for dipping. Chances are your friends will enjoy the healthier change, too.

I eat out at restaurants quite a bit and feel that I can't manage what I eat. Any suggestions?

Restaurants can actually be helpful to anyone trying to eat more healthily. You can't automatically go back for seconds, and you can control what is brought to the table. Do the obvious: select baked or broiled foods, order a salad, and request that extra rolls and butter be removed from the table. Avoid fried food and items smothered in cheese. Ask to split dessert with your dinner partner, or have a bowl of fresh fruit instead of a calorie-laden cake or pie. Anyone eating out more than once a week must be very thoughtful when ordering. If you can't make good choices or you continue to feel you eat too much when dining out, STOP DOING IT! Think ahead, pack a sandwich or eat at home, then go out.

I'm hungry all the time. How can I satisfy my hunger without overeating?

If you're hungry all the time, then you're probably not eating enough, or you aren't sitting down and taking enough time to enjoy a full meal. New mothers are often pressed for time, and lunch may be half a sandwich crammed in while you do the laundry. This kind of eating doesn't provide you with enough food or the satisfaction associated with eating a relaxed, pleasurable meal. Start taking the time to eat three meals a day plus snacks. Allow at least fifteen minutes for a meal.

If you're eating as much as you should based on my guidelines and you're still hungry, munch on low-fat snacks. See page 200 for some ideas. If you're eating enough and still losing weight faster than recommended for nursing mothers, you may need to talk to your doctor. Unsatisfied hunger can indicate medical problems.

I live with my mother, and she cooks too much. If I don't eat everything she makes, she gets mad at me. What can I do?

This can be a hard problem for someone trying to eat differently. The person doing the cooking often uses food to express affection.

If you refuse the food, it can be interpreted as a rejection of that person. Ask your mother for her help. Tell her she's a great cook but that since you've had the baby you're trying to eat a little differently: more fruits and vegetables, fewer fried foods, and only the amounts you feel you need. Then tell her the foods you want to stay away from and whatever other changes you plan to initiate, such as no second portions or no added gravy. Then stick to what you say. If one day you say you won't do this and the next day you do, she'll get a mixed message and you'll be right back where you started.

I keep cookies and chips around for my older children. How do I stop picking on them myself?

If you can't control yourself around snack foods that aren't very healthful, the only solution is to stop bringing them into the house. Tell your children about the change. Instead of keeping high-calorie snack foods around, make them special-occasion treats. You can take everybody out for a treat once a week or make a special coffee cake, bake a great homemade cake, or buy a specialty bakery cake. Freeze any leftovers so you won't be tempted to nibble. The point here is to not have ready-to-eat snack foods around that you can't resist.

My stepchildren visit on weekends and I always feel I have to make big fancy meals. How can I do this and watch what I eat?

First of all, you're probably going to be too tired to make big fancy meals once your new baby arrives. Your stepchildren need to have good, healthy food, but they don't need fancy or elabo- rate meals. The same foods that are good for you are good for your family. Meals should have at least two vegetables, a main dish, some starch, and perhaps some fruit for dessert. Try any of the ideas in the recipe section, or adapt your old family favorites using my healthier eating guidelines in chapter 10.

I'm a single mother and cooking for one is just too much. How can I get healthy meals?

When your baby is still on breast milk alone, it's hard to prepare big meals just for yourself. If this is your problem, try some of my ready-to-eat suggestions in chapter 10. Not eating good food is not an option for you.

SIX EATING STRATEGIES

Here are some simple eating strategies that can help you stick to your healthy new diet while you breastfeed—and, I hope, for all the years while you watch your new baby grow up.

1. Don't skip meals.
2. Try to eat in one place or eat only if sitting down (this helps me not to pick at food while I cook).
3. Don't keep troublesome foods in the house. Stock up on snacks that are good for you: yogurt, low-fat cheese sticks, vegetable soup, vegetables, salads, and fruit. Keep sliced vegetables on hand.
4. Ask your family, friends, or partner for help in eating better.
5. Incorporate healthy exercise into your life.
6. Chew your food well and eat slowly. This is a good habit, and if you do it, your kids are more likely to do it, too.

What should I weigh?

Use the Body Mass Index (BMI) on the following page to plot a desirable weight.

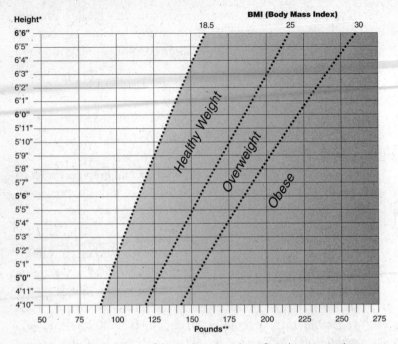

Find your weight on the bottom of the graph. Go straight up from that point until you come to the line that matches your height. Then look to find your weight group. The higher your BMI is over 25, the greater chance you may have of developing health problems.
*Without shoes.   **Without clothes.

Source: Weight Control Information Network
www.niddk.nih.gov/health/nutrit/nutrit.htm.

12

WHAT'S NEXT?

The first eleven chapters will aid in a healthy, satisfying breastfeeding and mothering experience. This chapter will give you the advice you need to eat well and feed yourself and your child after you stop breastfeeding. We live in a world with an abundance of food choices and information, and you will be faced with decisions that are much more complicated than your choice to nurse. After thirty years of experience as a dietitian and mother of two children, I have been asked almost every food- and nutrition-related question about women and raising a family. This chapter sums up what I think you need to know to feed yourself and your children as they grow.

FAMILY NUTRITION—WHAT TO PUT ON THE TABLE?

You might think nutrition professionals are inconsistent or confused about what to advise families to eat. We aren't. Sensational stories and headlines are produced by media outlets with the primary purpose of maintaining viewers and readers. News needs to be exciting, and most Americans obtain nutrition information from the media and not health professionals. In 2006, a $400 million study was published in the *Journal of the American Medical*

Association and is gathering huge press. The results of this eight-year, fifty-thousand-participant research project sponsored by the National Heart Lung and Blood Institute (NHLBI) concluded that the simple message to eat a low-fat diet would not protect against many serious illnesses. The results of this study were no surprise to nutrition professionals. Years ago we learned that the "all fat is bad" message was misguided. The full message is more complex and should include: reduce harmful fat (saturated and *trans*-fat); include the good fats (poly- and monounsaturated fat); eat whole grains, more fruits, and vegetables; control your weight; and be active every day.

The science of nutrition is always expanding. Don't be distracted by breaking studies in the media. What you feed your family is important and there is plenty of good science to offer you guidance. The following suggestions about what to serve at your table are based on years of experience as a dietitian and not on diet fads or trends. The Family Table should include the following foods:

Whole Grains: Every adult in the family needs three servings a day and children need one to three servings. See chapter 6 for serving sizes. (A serving for young children might be only one or two tablespoons for each year of life.) See page 193 for cooking suggestions.

Fats: "No fat" is the wrong message. Fat carries flavor and plant oils including olive, canola, soy, corn, sunflower, and peanut carry essential fatty acids that are good for you and your family. Soft margarines and salad dressings made with these oils should be part of your diet and your child's diet.

Vegetables: We are not eating enough. Vegetables can help with weight control and carry nutrients that fight disease. Potatoes are the most popular American vegetable, but unfortunately potatoes do not carry the same nutrition as more colorful vegetables like green beans and carrots. Potatoes should be lumped with other starchy foods such as pasta and rice.

Fruit: Everyone needs at least two servings a day. The portion sizes listed in chapter 6 are examples of serving sizes.

Protein: The best sources are lean and low in saturated fat. This includes poultry, fish, lean pork, eggs, nuts, and beans. Save fatty red meats for special occasions and ground beef only once, maybe twice, per week.

Milk: Dairy foods are the easiest way to get calcium. Low-fat choices carry the same calcium and protein as their whole-milk counterparts. Most of us need one to three servings daily. If you are not a milk drinker, get calcium from a supplement or read about alternate sources on pages 84 and 154.

I STILL NEED TO LOSE WEIGHT

Not all women lose weight while breastfeeding. If you're nearing the end of your nursing experience or have already stopped and want to lose more weight, you can probably be more aggressive in meeting your weight goals. Weight loss occurs only when there is a deficit of calories. Any diet will work if you stick to it, but in order to stay with a diet, the menu must be filling and satisfying. The food components that effect satiety include water, fiber, fat, protein, and liquids.

The Importance of Water—It's Different from What You May Think!

Research shows that over the course of one or two days a person will eat the same weight in food. If you eat the foods that weigh more and contain fewer calories, you will feel full while eating fewer calories. Foods that weigh more contain more water. Such foods include fruits, vegetables, yogurt, milk, soup, and so on.

While many women believe drinking a lot of water helps lose weight, Barbara Rolls, Ph.D., at the University of Pennsylvania has a different approach. She has found that water consumed alongside a meal empties out of the stomach quickly, preventing a sense of fullness, but when water is contained within a meal, people do feel full. To prove her point, she offered three different meals to a group of women and measured how much they ate. On one day she served a chicken-and-rice casserole, on another day chicken-and-rice casserole with water on the side, and on a third day chicken-and-rice casserole with ten ounces of water mixed in and served as a soup. Though the calories were the same in each meal, the soup eaters consumed 100 calories less and did not make up for it at other meals. This finding is significant because it allowed for a lower total calorie intake without hunger, and hunger is always the dieter's nemesis.

How to use water to your advantage:

- To help with satiety, eat foods that have a high water content: yogurt, soup, fruit, vegetables: foods that are literally "wet" to the touch.
- Don't give up on drinking water—just don't count on it as your sole weight-control strategy.
- Drinking water to replace soda is a good idea because it cuts calories.
- Under Resources you'll find a reference to Barbara Rolls's cookbook, called *Volumetrics*. It illustrates this water/weight principle deliciously.

Fiber

Doubling fiber from 15 to 30 grams can reduce calorie intake. High-fiber foods require more chewing, which slows the eating process and encourages us to eat less. Also, the fiber can absorb water and weigh more. Fiber may slow digestion and it may stimulate hormones that tell the brain to stop eating. Foods high in fiber weigh more, and larger portions can be eaten because high-fiber foods are lower in calories.

How to use fiber to your advantage:

- Eat at least three servings of whole grain food every day.
- Include a fruit or a vegetable or both at every meal.
- Include fruit or vegetables as part or all of your snack choices.

Protein

Proteins are filling, but choose wisely. To keep hunger pangs at bay, include protein at each meal. Good protein sources can come from the protein group listed on page 85 or from the dairy products listed in the milk group on page 83.

How to use protein to your advantage:

- At breakfast include an egg, Canadian bacon, a glass of low-fat milk, or a low-fat yogurt.
- At lunch or dinner include lean meats, chicken, fish, beans, or vegetarian "burgers."
- When really hungry and craving something "solid," consider a hard-boiled egg, or a slice of chicken, to fill you up.
- To keep calories low while eating protein, limit fried foods such as fried chicken or fish to once per week.
- Cheese, including cheddar, Swiss, American, Colby, and Muenster carry 100 calories per ounce, with about half of those calories coming from animal fat. I recommend a limit of one serving of regular cheese once per week for anyone trying to control weight. This includes cheese pizza, cheese casseroles, or a grilled cheese sandwich.

Fat

Reducing fat is one of the most effective ways to trim calories, but do not eliminate it. A no-fat diet does not work. It is not satisfying and many no-fat foods such as pretzels and crackers add lots of calories, but because they carry no "water weight," they are not likely to be filling. The fat from olive oil, canola oil, and other plant oils are good for your heart, and fat is essential for taste and satiety. Fat carries 45 calories in a teaspoon. There are three teaspoons in a tablespoon; a tablespoon of butter, olive oil, or any vegetable oil carries about 140 calories. Preparing two cups of green beans (100 calories) in two tablespoons of olive oil or butter will add at least 200 calories, for a total of 300 calories. Serve the same green beans with lemon or a butter spray and the calories will stay at 100.

How to use fat to your advantage:

- At least once, measure and observe what a teaspoon of margarine and olive oil look like. This will teach you how to gauge portion size.
- Most women should aim to keep their servings from the fat group to two portions per meal. Review what foods (and suggested portions) are in the fat group on page 89.
- When sautéing food, spray the pan with a spray oil that adds a fraction of the calories you would use, and add a teaspoon of olive or canola oil for flavor.

DON'T FORGET ABOUT CALORIES

I recommend regular meals containing protein, fruits, vegetables, and whole grains, because I have found that regular balanced meals allow individuals to control calories most effectively. No matter how you eat, if you want to lose weight, you must eat fewer calories than you burn, so never forget that; calories do count. The NHLBI recommends that women (not breastfeeding and not pregnant) needing to lose weight will have to reduce their calories by 500 to 1,000 calories each day to lose one to two pounds per week. A suggested calorie range for women wanting to lose weight is 1,000 to 1,200 calories per day and 1,200 to 1,600 for women who weigh 165 pounds or more or who exercise every day. Despite the NHLBI recommendations, I think 1,200 calories will be too low for most new mothers. I think most mothers will need at least 1,500 calories to meet the energy needs of raising children. Many mothers are up at night to tend to wakeful children and chasing kids during the day. Such women have energy demands that women without kids don't have.

How to use calories to your advantage:

- You should have a sense of the calorie content of the food groups. Such information is included in the description of each of the food groups in chapter 6.

- You can keep food records if you have the time, but if time is precious, I recommend that you limit the portions from the starch group to about 160 calories per meal and the fat group to about 90 calories.
- If you have favorite foods you order at fast-food or drive-thru restaurants, go online to their websites and learn how many calories you obtain in your favorite items. I once had a client who always ordered the coffee cake muffin at a popular drive-thru. She was completely ignorant of the fact that this one muffin contained 700 calories. She could have two egg sandwiches (at 310 each) for each muffin. Web addresses for popular restaurant chains are listed in the Resource section of this book.

SUCCESSFUL LOSERS

People do lose weight and keep it off permanently. James Hill, Ph.D., at the University of Colorado Health Sciences in Denver, Colorado, has created the National Weight Control Registry. Membership is now at five thousand and it includes people who have successfully lost sixty pounds and kept it off for five years. Here is what they do:

- Three-quarters of the registry members weigh themselves once per week.
- Some but not all members keep food diaries.
- Most eat five small meals each day (a good reason for family meals).
- Breakfast is never skipped.
- Less than 1 percent ate a low-carbohydrate diet.
- Most eat a low-fat, high-carbohydrate diet (carbohydrates come from fruit, vegetables, and dairy).
- Those who have lost the sixty pounds tend to exercise about an hour a day, or walk twelve thousand steps (five to six miles) per day.

- Many who are successful losers have tried and failed diets before.

PUTTING IT ALL TOGETHER

Our appetite and hunger are controlled by a complex system of checks and balances. If you eat too little, the stomach produces a hormone called ghrelin that increases hunger and calls for the body to eat. Our fat cells produce a hormone called leptin. This hormone is believed to sense when our fat storage is adequate; when the body has stored enough fat the brain is told to stop eating. For some of us this message system to decrease hunger is not as effective as it could be. Keeping ourselves well fed but not overfed may help this system of appetite control be more effective. As a new mother you have the perfect opportunity to put a permanent healthy eating plan into practice. Not only will your health and weight be in control, regular meals will foster healthy families as well. Healthy eating does not have to be complex, tedious, or depriving.

The following suggestions will help you control weight permanently.

- Eat three meals on most days and include breakfast. Have a schedule—try to stay within one hour of that schedule on most days, including weekends. This will prevent you from becoming hungry and give you the mental focus to make healthy food choices.
- Eat a fruit or a vegetable or both at every meal. These foods will help fill you up and they promote good nutrition.
- Include lean protein at every meal. Protein can come from food in the milk group such as a cup of milk in cereal or a yogurt, or it can come from foods in the protein group. Review the food groups in chapter 6.
- Eat enough at meals to feel satisfied but take second portions from the fruit, vegetable, protein, or milk group. To control

calories limit portions from the fat group and the starch group.

- Eat at a table and aim to allow at least fifteen minutes for eating.
- Choose snacks wisely. Your best snack choice will be "wet" foods. These carry fiber and water to help control appetite.
- Best snack choices:

All whole fruits including applesauce, whole fruit, fruit salad, canned fruit in juice or water. Limit juice to six ounces (because it contains no fiber and won't be as filling as whole fruit) and limit dried fruit to a quarter cup (because all the water weight has been removed and it won't be very filling, either).

All vegetables including vegetable soup, vegetable juice, and vegetable salad.

Low-fat calcium choices can include: skim and low-fat milk, yogurt, soy yogurt, soy milk, tofu, low-fat cottage cheese, skim-milk mozzarella cheese sticks, pudding made with low-fat milk.

Lean protein: When you are hungry, a food rich in protein can be very filling and, unlike chips or cookies, it doesn't lead to constant snacking. Good choices might include a hard-boiled egg, a slice of deli ham or Canadian bacon, a slice of turkey, or a veggie burger.

In most cases I recommend you eat starchy or dry foods with meals and not as snacks, to better control your portions. Such foods include pasta, bread, rice, noodles, crackers, chips, cookies, and so on. If you do eat these foods between meals, limit your servings to about 100-calorie portions. If you choose from my suggested list, you get the foods that are more nutritious and you eat less because these are foods your body and appetite tend to self-limit. Given a bag of chips, you might eat the whole bag. Given a bag of apples, you are likely to stop after one apple.

Exercise increases the rate at which we burn calories and acts as an appetite suppressant, not a stimulant. Adult women should exercise the equivalent of thirty minutes of walking each day. I recommend you aim for daily exercise. This way, if you fail (and I often do), you will end up walking four or five times a week. Proper diet must accompany your exercise plan in order to keep weight in check. A thirty-minute walk may burn only 150 calories, half the number of calories in a small sandwich. Exercise is very important, but my experience has been that it is most effective in its ability to keep weight off and in preventing weight gain over time. Don't count on exercise alone to lose weight unless you are extremely active—food choices matter for most of us!

Special Food Consideration

Heart disease, high blood pressure, and diabetes are all conditions that increase in risk with age and affect about ninety million Americans. While the above eating guidelines will help prevent weight gain, which exacerbates these conditions, there is even more you can do. Ongoing nutrition studies have found that certain foods are particularly beneficial to promoting good health and preventing disease. The following suggestions will help you truly balance your diet for a healthier future:

Try to eat fish twice a week. (Read about fish safety on page 145.)

Try eating "vegetarian" a few times per week.

Include a small amount of nuts at least three times per week or use nuts as a protein source at meals more often. Examples include a peanut butter sandwich instead of a hamburger or a salad with nuts in it instead of cheese.

Limit alcohol—daily moderate intake is defined as one drink for women and two for men.

Choose at least three of your starches as whole grain; for most families choosing a breakfast cereal and whole grain bread is the easiest way to do this. Of course frozen whole wheat waffles are popular, too.

Have fun trying new food!

HOW TO HELP YOUR CHILDREN

Observation, discussion, and education have led me to believe that most of the family meal habits, structure, and attitudes are established in the first eighteen months of a child's life. The way you introduce food, how you set up the feeding environment, and your role as a parent are developed earlier than you may have expected. The recommendations that follow are intended to help you lay the foundation for a lifetime of happy, pleasant meals. There are plenty of baby-feeding books that will tell you what to feed and when. This section is about developing a healthy food environment for the purpose of avoiding the struggles so many parents face. The following suggestions are made based on the questions I am asked over and over again about feeding kids.

The Importance of the Family Table

I am certain that everyone reading this book is not only concerned about nutrition but also the emotional well-being of their children. There is a simple and effective solution to proper nutrition and emotional security. It is called "the family meal." The family meal provides an opportunity to connect as a family. It helps both children and parents regulate their food intake and feel secure. Demands of jobs plus social and community commitments tear at this age-old tradition, but do not give it up lightly; doing so can undermine your family.

As you develop your family rituals and routines, please include the importance of the family meal and the family structure. By fifteen to eighteen months of age, young children should be on a predictable three-meal-per-day schedule with planned snacks offered in between. The secondary benefits of regularly scheduled meals include better nutrition and, as I will explain, even weight control. It may seem like the teen years are a lifetime away, but they will be here before you know it and the way you parent and feed your infant impacts your child's behavior when they are older.

A YMCA parent and teen survey has found that the number one concern reported by teens was not having enough time with their parents. In another report put out by the White House Council of Economic Advisors, it was found that teens who eat dinner with their families five times in a week were less likely to smoke, drink, use drugs, or be involved in early sexual activity. If family meals can do this much good, they are worth the trouble.

Childhood Overweight and Obesity

Obesity is now considered the number one health risk to our children's quality of life as they grow older. Some health professionals rate it higher than drug abuse and smoking; it is an enormous concern. Most Americans blame cable television, the Internet, video games, and fast-food restaurants as the major contributors to obesity in our children. I think these are actually the symptoms and not the causes. There is nothing wrong with a child playing video games or working on the Internet (as long as the content is appropriate). These activities burn as many if not more calories than book reading, an activity that we encourage. My concern regarding this technology is twofold: Is there eating going on while these activities are happening? And are these activities occurring at the exclusion of family time and daily exercise? This is a parenting issue and not a nutrition issue. It is very important as you create your family feeding traditions to understand how very important you are to your children and how important it is that you spend time with your children. You might think it is odd to state the obvious need for kids to spend time with parents, but as your children get older you will find there are many, many obligations that will work against family time. If families follow these simple suggestions most of the time, childhood obesity can be avoided.

Have Regularly Scheduled Meals

Most parents are surprised when I tell them it is not their job to make a child eat. A parent's job is to serve wholesome food in a calm and peaceful environment. To be successful at family meals, have a meal and snack structure. Children thrive on routine and it will make them feel secure knowing they do not have to worry about when they will eat next. Children can regulate their food portions when they know that food will be offered in a predictable manner.

Serve a Variety of Food—but Don't Force Anybody to Eat Anything

Many researchers have studied how children self-regulate. Given a schedule and access to good food, children will eat what they need at a meal. Dr. Nancy Butte has found that offering children a variety of flavors in the first two years of life can lead to the better acceptance of new and more varied foods later on. Dr. Leanne Birch has found that children must be offered a new food five to ten times before it becomes familiar. Do not assume a child does not like a food just because he refuses it once. Try, try again! Don't assume just because YOU do not like a food that your child won't, either.

Don't Be Overcontrolling

It is not your job to determine how much food your child needs to eat. Ask yourself if you would like it if your spouse insisted you eat a food that you found highly suspicious, or refused to allow you to eat a favorite food until you ate a dreaded food. If such tactics encouraged healthy enthusiastic eaters, I would encourage them, but they do not. Instead, they turn meals into a battleground. Ellyn Satter, M.S.W., has found in her research that parents who are overcontrolling in the area of food teach a child self-doubt and probably create a pickier eater. On the other hand, children who are trusted to eat what they need learn responsibility and have better self-esteem. I highly recommend Ellyn Satter's book, *Child of Mine*. It is one of my favorite family feeding books and is listed in Resources.

Child Food Safety

Avoid serving hard round foods; they can cause choking. This includes hard candies, hot dogs, and carrots. Sitting down while eating will allow for safer meals because children will be more focused on eating and chewing.

Television and Your Child

Excessive television watching is associated with feelings of isolation and obesity. When kids are old enough to watch TV, the American Academy of Pediatrics recommends a limit of 2 hours per day. I suggest no TV during the week and no TV in the bedroom.

Suggestions for Coping with Fast-Food Meals

Fast-food eating is a reality for some families. If you do it only once per week, enjoy what you want, but if you eat fast food more than once a week, read my suggestions below about meal choices.

- Limit sweets to one per meal such as one soda or one dessert.
- Limit fried food to one time per meal: an order of fries or a fried sandwich.
- Include a fruit or a vegetable (you may have to pack one).
- Keep portions child-size—choose regular-size sandwiches, not those described as "double," "triple," or "grande."
- Include a small yogurt or milk if your child is still hungry.

PUTTING IT ALL TOGETHER FOR KIDS

The following suggestions will help your kids:

- Serve balanced meals and let your child eat what she chooses.
- The definition of balanced is: something from the protein group, at least one serving from the vegetable group or fruit

group, or both. Include at least one food from the starch group, maybe two food items. In addition, something from the milk group can be included. Include something from the fat group. If you have available a variety of foods, at least three to five items, and you serve them at the table, you are doing what you need to nourish your child. Then, trust your child to eat what she needs.

- Have a three-meal schedule and offer a snack between meals. Do not become frustrated or alarmed if your child eats voraciously at one meal and picks at the next—this is normal.
- Combine favorite foods (most kids like bread, pasta, and noodles) with new foods, such as a new or less popular vegetable.
- Serve only one new or unpopular food at a time.
- Make meals pleasant. Don't discuss who is eating what at the table. Save discussions about meal routines when meals are not being eaten. Table manners, attitude, and general behavior should be discussed as it happens. If mealtime is a battle zone, step back and figure out what is wrong.
- Serve child-size portions of dessert regularly so children do not learn to covet these items. Once a day is fine for most kids.
- Have designated eating areas. Sit down and join your children when they eat. As your children get older, discourage eating while watching TV or playing video games or working on the computer. Keep eating a mindful activity; otherwise hundreds of calories can be consumed thoughtlessly and not because of hunger. If you make this a family rule early on, it will be the norm.
- Each child should be active every day. Support your child in being active. Children are motivated to be active 100 percent by fun. Give them active toys, jump rope, bouncy balls, and so on, and set a good example yourself.

As you end your nursing experience, you move toward the beginning of a roller-coaster ride called parenting. None of us do it perfectly—we just do the best we can. Breastfeeding was your first smart choice. Trust your instincts but take guidance from others as well. I hope the guidelines suggested in this book will make your job easier. May you have many happy, healthy meals with your new baby.

It's always exciting to hear from people who read my books. If you have a comment about the book or want to share an experience, I'd like to hear from you.

Write to Eileen Behan at Ballantine Books, 1745 Broadway, New York, NY 10019.

ORGANIZATIONS AND WEBSITES THAT MAY BE OF HELP TO NEW MOMS

Allergies

The Food Allergy and Anaphylaxis Network
www.foodallergy.org

American Academy of Allergy, Asthma, and Immunology
www.aaaai.org

Vegetarian Nutrition

Vegetarian Resource Group
www.vrg.org

North American Vegetarian Society
www.navs-online.org

Child Health

Academy of Family Physicians
www.familydoctor.org
www.aafp.org

American Academy of Pediatrics
www.aap.org

Diabetes

American Diabetes Association
www.diabetes.org

National Diabetes Information Clearinghouse
http://diabetes.niddk.nih.gov/

Breast Pumps

If you are having trouble with your pump or have questions, call the La Leche
League or contact a lactation consultant. Several of the websites listed below
offer very good information about breastfeeding pumps and other breastfeeding-
related issues.

Medela breast pump manufacturer
www.medela.com

Ameda breast pump
www.hollister.com

Bailey Medical Engineering
www.baileymed.com

Easy Expression Hands-Free Bustier
www.easyexpressionproducts.com

Breast Pump.com, Inc., foot-powered breast pump
www.breastpump.com

Whittlestone Breast Pump
www.whittlestone.com

Lactation Consultants and Organizations

International Childbirth Education Association
www.icea.org/info.htm

International Lactation Consultant Association
www.ilca.org

Lactation Institute and Breastfeeding Clinic
www.lactationinstitute.org

Wellstart International Corporate Headquarters
www.wellstart.org

La Leche League International
www.lalecheleague.com

Nutritionists

To find a professional nutritionist, go to the American Dietetic Association website at: www.eatright.org and click "find a nutrition professional."

Women's Issues

Maternal and Child Health Resources
www.mchirc.net

National Women's Health Information Center
www.4woman.gov

NUTRITION RESOURCES/NEWSLETTERS

Environmental Nutrition
www.environmentalnutrition.com

Mayo Clinic Health Letter
www.mayohealth.org

Tufts University, Health and Nutrition Letter
www.healthletter.tufts.edu

University of California, Berkeley Wellness Letter
1-800-829-9080

Center for Science in the Public Interest
Nutrition Action Health Letter
www.cspinet.org

FAVORITE BOOKS

Child of Mine: Feeding with Love and Good Sense by Ellyn Satter (Bull Publishing, 2000)
Eat, Drink and Be Healthy by Walter Willett (Free Press, 2002)
Stretching by Bob Anderson (Shelter Publications, Inc., 1980)
The Nursing Mother's Companion by Kathleen Huggins (La Leche League, 2005)
Volumetrics Eating Plan by Barbara Rolls (Morrow Cookbooks, 2005)
Womanly Art of Breastfeeding (La Leche League, 2004)

FAST-FOOD WEB RESOURCES

Arby's
www.arbys.com

Burger King
www.burgerking.com

Dairy Queen
www.dairyqueen.com

Domino's Pizza
www.dominos.com

Dunkin Donuts
www.dunkindonuts.com

Jack in the Box
www.jackinthebox.com

KFC
www.kfc.com

McDonald's
www.mcdonalds.com

Starbucks
www.starbucks.com

Subway
www.subway.com

Taco Bell
www.tacobell.com

Wendy's
www.wendys.com

REFERENCES

Breastfeeding: A Guide for the Medical Profession, 6th ed., by Ruth A. Lawrence and Robert M. Lawrence (C. Mosby, Inc., 2005).

Nutrition During Lactation. Subcommittee of Nutrition During Lactation of the National Academy of Sciences. Washington, D.C., 1991 Report, Institute of Medicine.

Krause's Food, Nutrition and Diet Therapy, by L. K. Mahan and S. Escott-Stump (New York: Elsevier, 2004).

The bibliography that follows lists the references for additional research used in each chapter.

Chapter 1

Abbott Laboratories (2003). New data show U.S. breastfeeding rates at all-time recorded high. www.ross.com, search: 2003 Breastfeeding Rates. Accessed 2/1/06.

Chapman JJ (1985). Concerns of breastfeeding mothers from birth to 4 months. *Nursing Research* 34(6):374–77.

Elias MF (1986). Sleep/wake patterns of breastfed infants the first two years of life. *Pediatrics* 77(3):322–29.

Grummer-Strawn LM (2004). Does breastfeeding protect against pediatric overweight? Analysis of longitudinal data from the Centers for Disease Control and Prevention Pediatric Nutrition Surveillance System. *Pediatrics* 113(2): e81–86.

Harder T (2005). Duration of breastfeeding and risk of overweight: A meta-analysis. *American Journal of Epidemiology* 162(5):397–403.

Healthy People 2000: National Health Promotion and Disease Prevention Objectives. DHHS Pub. No. (PHS) 91-50213. Washington, D.C.: U.S. Department of Health and Human Services, U.S. Government Printing Office.

Howie PW (1990). Protective effect of breastfeeding against infection. *British Medical Journal* 300:11–16.

Labbok M (1987). Does breastfeeding protect against malocclusion? *American Journal of Preventive Medicine* 3:227–32.

Lee K (2000). Crying and behavior pattern in breast- and formula-fed infants. *Early Human Development* 58(2):133–40.

Li R (2003). Prevalence of breastfeeding in the United States: The 2001 National Immunization Survey. *Pediatrics* 113(3Pt 1):626–27.

Lucas A (1998). Crying, fussing and colic behavior in breast- and bottle-fed infants. *Early Human Development* 53(1):9–18.

Mortensen EL (2002). The association between duration of breastfeeding and adult intelligence. *Journal of the American Medical Association* 287(22):2946.

Pinella T (1993). Help me make it through the night: Behavioral entrainment of breastfed infants' sleep patterns. *Pediatrics* 91(6):883–85.

Singhal A (2004). Early origins of cardiovascular disease: Is there a unifying hypothesis? *Lancet* 363(9421):1642–45.

Stuebe AM (2005). Duration of lactation and incidence of type 2 diabetes. *Journal of the American Medical Association* 294(20):2601–10.

Chapter 2

Allen LH (1994). Maternal micronutrient malnutrition: Effects on breast milk and infant nutrition, and priorities for intervention. *Science News* (11):21–24.

American Academy of Pediatrics Committee on Nutrition (2004). *Pediatric Nutrition Handbook,* 5th ed. Elk Grove Village, Ill.: American Academy of Pediatrics.

Dietary Reference Intakes (2004). The Food and Nutrition Board of the Institute of Medicine, National Academy of Sciences. www.iom.edu/report.

Picciano MF (2003). Pregnancy and lactation: Physiological adjustments, nutritional requirements and the role of dietary supplements. *Journal of Nutrition* 133(6):1997s–2002s.

Spin the bottle: How to pick a multivitamin (January/February 2003). *Nutrition Action Health Letter.* www.cspinet.org/nah/01_03/spin.pdf.

Thomas MR (1980). The effects of vitamin C, vitamin B_6, vitamin B_{12}, folic acid, riboflavin, and thiamine on the breast milk and maternal status of well-nourished women at 6 months postpartum. *American Journal of Clinical Nutrition* 33:2151–56.

Chapter 3

American Academy of Pediatrics Committee on Nutrition (2004). *Pediatric Nutrition Handbook,* 5th ed. Elk Grove Village, Ill.: American Academy of Pediatrics.

Anderson DM (1985). Vitamin E and C concentrations in human milk with maternal mega dosing. *Journal of the American Dietetic Association* 85:715–17.

Bolton RA (1990). Fluoride supplementation of the breastfed infant. *Journal of the American Medical Association* 263(16):2170.

Dietary Reference Intake for Calcium, Phosphorous, Magnesium, Vitamin D, and Fluoride (1997). Dietary Reference Intakes for Thiamin, Riboflavin, Niacin, Vitamin B_6, Folate, Vitamin B_{12}, Pantothenic Acid, Biotin, and Choline (1998). Dietary Reference Intakes for Vitamin A, Vitamin K, Arsenic, Boron, Chromium, Copper, Iodine, Iron, Manganese, Molybdenum, Nickel, Silicon, Vanadium, and Zinc (2000). Dietary Reference Intakes for Vitamin C, Vitamin E, Selenium, and Carotenoids (2000). Dietary Reference Intakes for Energy, Carbohydrate, Fiber, Fat, Fatty Acids, Cholesterol, Protein, and Amino Acids (macronutrients) (2002). Dietary Reference Intakes for Water, Potassium, Sodium, Chloride, and Sulfate (2004). Food and Nutrition Board, Institute of Medicine, National Academy of Sciences.

Hambidge KM (2003). Zinc, low birth weight, and breastfeeding. *Pediatrics* 112:1419–20.

Krebs NF (2002). Zinc and breastfed infants: If and when is there a risk of deficiency? *Advanced Experimental Biology* 503:69–75.

National Academics Press. The complete dietary reference intake reports listed above including tolerable upper intake levels can be accessed at www.nap.edu.

National Research Council (1989). *Recommended Dietary Allowances,* 10th ed. Washington, D.C.: National Academy Press.

West KD (1976). Influence of vitamin B_6 intake on the content of the vitamin in human milk. *American Journal of Clinical Nutrition* 29:961–69.

Chapter 4

Dusdieker PJ (1990). Prolonged maternal fluid supplementation in breastfeeding. *Pediatrics* 86:737–40.

Ludwig DS (1999). High glycemic index foods, overeating, and obesity. Electronic article. *Pediatrics* 103(3):e26. www.pediatrics.org/cgi/content/full/103/3/e26.

National Weight Control Registry. www.uchsc.edu/nutrition/WyattJortberg/nwcr.htm.

Stumbo PJ (1985). Water intakes of lactating women. *American Journal of Clinical Nutrition* 42:870–76.

Chapter 5

Brewer MM (1989). Postpartum changes in maternal weight and body fat deposits in lactating vs. nonlactating women. *American Journal of Clinical Nutrition* 49:259–65.

Butte NF (2005). Energy requirements during pregnancy and lactation. *Public Health Nutrition* 8(7A):1010–27.

Butte NF (2001). Energy requirements of lactating women derived from doubly labeled water and milk energy output. *Journal of Nutrition* 131:53–58.

Butte NF (2000). Dieting and exercise in overweight, lactating women. *New England Journal of Medicine* 342(7):502–3.

Butte NF (1984). Effect of maternal diet and body composition on lactational performance. *American Journal of Clinical Nutrition* 39:296–306.

Dewey KG (1993). Maternal weight-loss patterns during prolonged lactation. *American Journal of Clinical Nutrition* 58(2):162–66.

Haick LN (2001). Postpartum weight loss and infant feeding. *Journal of the American Board of Family Practice* 14(2):85–94.

Illingworth PJ (1985). Diminution in energy expenditure during lactation. *British Medical Journal* 292:1016–17.

Janney CA (1997). Lactation and weight retention. *American Journal of Clinical Nutrition* 66(5):1116–24.

Kaitschuck GK (1991, May). Breastfeeding and losing weight. *American Baby* 32.

Kramer FM (1993). Breastfeeding reduces maternal lower-body fat. *Journal of the American Dietetic Association* 93(4):429–33.

Lovelady CA (2000). The effect of weight loss in overweight, lactating women on the growth of their infants. *New England Journal of Medicine* 342(7):449–53.

Manning-Dalton C (1983). The effect of lactation on energy and protein composition, postpartum weight change and body composition of well-nourished North American women. *Nutrition Research* 3:293–308.

Manson JE (1995). Body weight and mortality among women. *New England Journal of Medicine* 333(11):677–85.

McCrory MA (2001). Does dieting during lactation put infant at risk? *Nutrition Reviews* 59(1pt1):18–21.

Mokdad AH (2003). Prevalence of obesity, diabetes, and obesity-related health risk factors, 2001. *Journal of the American Medical Association* 289(1):76–79.

Ohlin A (1996). Factors related to body weight changes during and after pregnancy: The Stockholm Pregnancy and Weight Development Study. *Obesity Research* 4(3):271–76.

Ohlin A (1994). Trends in eating patterns, physical activity and socio-demographic factors in relation to postpartum body weight development. *British Journal of Nutrition* 71(4):457–70.

Ohlin A (1990). Maternal body weight development after pregnancy. *International Journal of Obesity* 14(2):159–73.

O'Toole ML (2003). Structured diet and physical activity prevent postpartum weight retention. *Journal of Women's Health* 12(10):991–98.

Rexrode KM (1997). A prospective study of body mass index, weight change and risk of stroke in women. *Journal of the American Medical Association* 277(19):1539–45.

Rooney BL (2002). Excess pregnancy weight gain and long-term obesity: One decade later. *Obstetrics and Gynecology* 100(2):245–52.

Strode MA (1986). Effects of short-term calorie restriction on lactational performance of well-nourished women. *Acta Paediatrica Scandinavica* 75:222–29.

Willett WC (1995). Weight, weight change, and coronary heart disease in women: Risk within the "normal" range. *Journal of the American Medical Association* 273(6):461–65.

Chapter 6

Alfenas RC and Mattes RD (2005). Influence of glycemic index/load on glycemic response, appetite, and food intake in healthy humans. *Diabetes Care* 28(9):2123–29.

Bravata DM and Sanders L (2003). Efficacy and safety of low-carbohydrate diets: A systematic review. *Journal of the American Medical Association* 289:1837–50.

Doberne K and Heinig A (2004). Weight loss during lactation: Are low-carbohydrate diets a good choice? *Journal of Human Lactation* 20(3):341–42.

Zemel M (2002). Dietary calcium and dairy products accelerate weight and fat loss during energy restriction in obese adults. *American Journal of Clinical Nutrition* 275(suppl):342s–343s.

Chapter 7

ACOG Committee Opinion (2002). Exercise during pregnancy and the lactation period. *International Journal of Gynecology and Obstetrics* 77(1):79–81.

Baby Jogger Guidelines (1991). Letter to the editor. *The Physician and Sportsmedicine* 19(2):34.

Dewey KG (1998). Effects of maternal caloric restriction and exercise during lactation. *Journal of Nutrition* 128(2 suppl):386s–389s.

Dewey KG (1994). A randomized study of the effects of aerobic exercise by lactating women on breast-milk volume and composition. *New England Journal of Medicine* 330(7):449–53.

Larson-Meyer DE (2002). Effect of postpartum exercise on mothers and their offspring: A review of the literature. *Obesity Research* 10(8):841–53.

Lovelady, CA (1990). Lactation performance of exercising women. *American Journal of Clinical Nutrition* 52:103–9.

McCrory MA (1999). Randomized trial of the short-term effects of dieting compared with dieting plus aerobic exercise on lactation performance. *American Journal of Clinical Nutrition* 69(5):959–67.

Pacelli LC (1990). Parent-infant workouts: More harm than help? *The Physician and Sportsmedicine* 18(6):135–43.

Schelkon PH (1991). Exercise and breastfeeding mothers. *The Physician and Sportsmedicine* 19(4):109–16.

Chapter 8

Gladen BC (2000). Pubertal growth and development and prenatal and lactational exposure to polychlorinated biphenyls and dichlorodiphenyl dichloroethene. *Journal of Pediatrics* 136(4):490–96.

Grassi D (2005). Short-term administration of dark chocolate is followed by a significant increase in insulin sensitivity and a decrease in blood pressure in healthy persons. *American Journal of Clinical Nutrition* 81(3):611–14.

Jacobson JL (2003). Prenatal exposure to polychlorinated biphenyls and attention at school age. *Journal of Pediatrics* 143(6):780–88.

Jacobson JL (2002). Breastfeeding and gender as moderators of teratogenic effects on cognitive development. *Neurotoxicology Teratology* 24(3):349–58.

Little RE (1989). Maternal alcohol use during breastfeeding and infant mental and motor development at one year. *New England Journal of Medicine* 321:425–30.

Lovelady CA (1999). Weight change during lactation does not alter the concentrations of chlorinated organic contaminants in breast milk of women with low exposure. *Journal of Human Lactation* 15(4):307–15.

Lust K (1996). Maternal intake of cruciferous vegetables and other foods and colic symptoms in exclusively breastfed infants. *Journal of the American Dietetic Association* 96:47–48.

Mennella JA (2001). Regulation of milk intake after exposure to alcohol in mothers' milk. *Alcoholism: Clinical and Experimental Research* (4):590–3.

Mennella JA (1991). Maternal diet alters the sensory qualities of human milk and the nursling's behavior. *Pediatrics* 88(4):737–44.

Mennella JA (1991). The transfer of alcohol to human milk. *New England Journal of Medicine* 325:981–85.

Munoz LM (1988). Coffee consumption as a factor in iron-deficiency anemia among pregnant women and their infants in Costa Rica. *American Journal of Clinical Nutrition* 48:645–51.

Resman BH (1977). Breastmilk distribution of threobromine from chocolate. *The Journal of Pediatrics* 91(3):477–80.

Rogan WJ (1987). Polychlorinated biphenyls and dichlorodiphenyl dichloroethene in human milk: Effects on growth, morbidity and duration of lactation. *American Journal of Public Health* 77:1294–97.

Schardt D (2004, June). Farmed salmon under fire. *Nutrition Action Health Letter*, p 9–11.

Chapter 9

American Diabetes Association (2004). Nutrition principles and recommendations in diabetes. *Diabetes Care* 27(S1):36s–46s.

Blenning CE (2005). An approach to the postpartum office visit. *American Family Physician.* 72:2491–98.

Butte NF (1987). Milk composition of insulin-dependent diabetic women. *Journal of Pediatric Gastroenterology and Nutrition* 6:936–37.

Chandra RK (1987). Maternal dietary engineering reduces the incidence of allergic eczema. *Breastfeeding Abstracts* 7(7):1.

Cheruku SR (2002). Higher maternal plasma docosahexaenoic acid during pregnancy is associated with more mature neonatal sleep-state patterning. *American Journal of Clinical Nutrition* 76:608–13.

Clyne PS and Kulczycki, A (1991). Human breast milk contains bovine IgG, relationship to infant colic? *Pediatrics* 87(4):439–44.

Fahraeus L, Karson-Cohn O, and Wallentin L (1985). Plasma lipoprotein including high-density lipoprotein subfractions during normal pregnancy. *Obstetrics and Gynecology* 66: 468–72.

Gielen AC (1991). Maternal employment during the postpartum period: Effects on initiation and continuation of breastfeeding. *Pediatrics* 87:298–305.

Harris W (1984). Will dietary omega-3 fatty acids change composition of human milk? *American Journal of Clinical Nutrition* 40:780–87.

Jakobsson I (1983). Cow's milk proteins cause infantile colic in breastfed infants. *Pediatrics* 71(2):268.

Jakobsson I (1978, August). Cow's milk as a cause of infantile colic in breastfed infants. *The Lancet,* 437–39.

Knopp RH (1985). Effect of postpartum lactation on lipoproteins, lipids and apoproteins. *Journal of Clinical Endocrinology and Metabolism* 60:542–47.

Lust K (1996). Maternal intake of cruciferous vegetables and other foods and colic symptoms in exclusively breastfed infants. *Journal of the American Dietetic Association* 96:47–48.

Martin JA (2004). Preliminary births for 2004: Infant and maternal health. *National Center for Statistics.* www.cdc.gov/nch. Accessed 2/13/06.

Mellies MJ (1978). Effects of varying maternal dietary cholesterol and phytosterol in lactating women and their infants. *American Journal of Clinical Nutrition* 37:1347–54.

Popkin BM (2006). A new proposed guidance system for beverage consumption in the United States. *American Journal of Clinical Nutrition* 83:529–42.

Singhal A (2004). Breast milk feeding and lipoprotein profile in adolescents born preterm: Follow-up of a prospective randomized study. *Lancet* 363(9421): 1571–78.

Steube AM (2005). Duration of lactation and incidence of type 2 diabetes. *Journal of the American Medical Association* 294(20):2601–10.

3 in 10 mothers gave birth by C-section in 2004: Sharp, continuing rise defies best evidence and best practice. http://maternitywise.org/cesarean_response.html. Accessed 2/13/06.

Chapter 12

American Academy of Pediatrics (2001). Committee on Public Education: Children, adolescents, and television. *Pediatrics* 107(2):423–26.

Anderson CA (2006). Dietary modification and CVD prevention: A matter of fat. *Journal of the American Medical Association* 295(6):693–95.

Beresford SA (2006). Low-fat dietary pattern and risk of colorectal cancer: The Women's Health Inititive Randomized Controlled Dietary Modification Trial. *Journal of the American Medical Association* 295(6):643–54.

Birch L (1998). Development of eating behaviors among children and adolescents. *Pediatrics* 101(3 pt 2):539–49.

Butte N, Cobb K, Dwyer J, Graney L, Heird W, and Richard K (2004). The start-healthy feeding guidelines for infants and toddlers. *Journal of the American Dietetic Association* 104(3):442–54.

Buzdar AU (2006). Dietary modification and risk of breast cancer. *Journal of the American Medical Association* 295(6):691–92.

Howard BV (2006). Low-fat dietary pattern and risk of cardiovascular disease: The Women's Health Initiative Randomized Controlled Dietary Modification Trial. *Journal of the American Medical Association* 295(6):655–66.

Jackson M (2006, February 12). Repeat after me: "Welcome home, dear." *Boston Sunday Globe,* G1 and G7.

National Center on Addiction and Abuse at Columbia University (CASA). www.CASAFamilyDay.org. Accessed 6/6/06.

National Weight Control Registry. www.uchsc.edu/nutriton/WyattJortberg/nwcr.htm.

Prentice RL (2006). Low-fat dietary pattern and risk of invasive breast cancer: The Women's Health Initiative Randomized Controlled Dietary Modification Trial. *Journal of the American Medical Association* 295(6):629–42.

Reilly JJ (2005). Early life risk factors for obesity in childhood: Cohort study. *British Medical Journal* 330(7504):1357. Epub 2005, May 20.

Rolls B (1999). Water incorporated into a food but not served with a food decreases energy intake in lean women. *American Journal of Clinical Nutrition* 70:448–55.

Satter EM (1996). Internal regulation and the evolution of normal growth as the basis for prevention of obesity in children. *Journal of the American Dietetic Association* 96(9):860–64.

Talking with teens: The YMCA parent and teen survey final report. www.ymca.net/presrm/research/teensurvey.htm.

White House Council of Economic Advisers (2000). Teens and their parents in the twenty-first century: An examination of trends in teen behavior and the role of parental involvement. gov/wh/eop/cea/html/teens_paper_final.pdf.

INDEX

ABOUT THE AUTHOR

EILEEN BEHAN, R.D., is a member of the American Dietetic Association (ADA) and a registered dietitian. She has twenty-five years of experience working with individuals and families. Eileen trained as a dietitian at the Brigham and Women's Hospital in Boston, and completed the ADA adult weight-management program. She has worked for the Veterans Administration in Boston, the Harvard School of Public Health, and the Seacoast Family Practice in Exeter. Behan has published seven books including the bestselling *Eat Well, Lose Weight, While Breastfeeding.* Her other books include: *Microwave Cooking for Your Baby and Child; The Pregnancy Diet; Meals that Heal for Babies, Toddlers, and Children; Cooking Well for the Unwell; Fit Kids;* and *Therapeutic Nutrition: A Guide to Patient Education.* She has written for the *Washington Post, Newsweek, Parents* magazine, *Parenting,* and the Tufts University Nutrition Newsletter. She is a frequent lecturer on family nutrition and has been a contributor to the respected online health resource, WebMD. Behan has appeared on numerous television programs to discuss nutrition including CNN, CNBC, and the *Today Show.* She lives in the seacoast with her husband and two children.